OLIVIER DE SCHUTTER, HUGH FRAZER,
ANNE-CATHERINE GUIO
AND ERIC MARLIER

THE ESCAPE
FROM POVERTY

Breaking the Vicious Cycles
Perpetuating Disadvantage

POLICY PRESS **SHORTS** RESEARCH

First published in Great Britain in 2023 by

Policy Press, an imprint of
Bristol University Press
University of Bristol
1–9 Old Park Hill
Bristol
BS2 8BB
UK
t: +44 (0)117 374 6645
e: bup-info@bristol.ac.uk

Details of international sales and distribution partners are available at
policy.bristoluniversitypress.co.uk

British Library Cataloguing in Publication Data
A catalogue record for this book is available from the British Library

ISBN 978-1-4473-7060-4 hardcover
ISBN 978-1-4473-7062-8 ePub
ISBN 978-1-4473-7061-1 ePdf

Cover design: Bristol University Press
Front cover image: Benoît Lanscotte/LISER
Bristol University Press and Policy Press use environmentally
responsible print partners.
Printed and bound in Great Britain by CPI Group (UK) Ltd,
Croydon, CR0 4YY

This book is dedicated to the memory of
Tony Atkinson and Fintan Farrell, who, throughout
their lives, actively and relentlessly fought against
poverty and inequality and for social justice
across Europe and around the world.

Contents

List of abbreviations

ARC–CRSA	Alternate Report Coalition – Children's Rights South Africa
CESCR	Committee on Economic, Social and Cultural Rights
COFACE	Confederation of Family Organisations in the European Union
CPRC	Chronic Poverty Research Centre
EAPN	European Anti-Poverty Network
ECEC	early childhood education and care
EMCO	Employment Committee
ESPAN	European Social Policy Analysis Network
EU	European Union
EU–SILC	European Union Statistics on Income and Living Conditions
FAO	Food and Agriculture Organization
GDP	gross domestic product
HBSC	Health Behaviour in School-Aged Children
HLPE	High-Level Panel of Experts on Food Security and Nutrition
HLPF	High-Level Political Forum
IBRD	International Bank for Reconstruction and Development
IGPP	inter-generational perpetuation of poverty
ILO	International Labour Organization
IMF	International Monetary Fund

IPCC	Intergovernmental Panel on Climate Change
LEAP	Livelihood Empowerment Against Poverty
MENA	Middle East and North Africa
OECD	Organisation for Economic Co-operation and Development
OHCHR	Office of the High Commissioner for Human Rights
PACE	Parliamentary Assembly of the Council of Europe
PISA	Programme for International Student Assessment
pp	percentage points
PPP	purchasing power parity
PUCL	People's Union for Civil Liberties
SDG	Sustainable Development Goal
SPC	Social Protection Committee
SPPM	Social Protection Performance Monitor
UK	United Kingdom
UN	United Nations
UNDP	United Nations Development Programme
UNESCO	United Nations Educational, Scientific and Cultural Organization
UNICEF	United Nations International Children's Emergency Fund
US	United States
US$	United States dollar
VAT	value added tax
WHO	World Health Organization

About the authors

Olivier De Schutter is Professor at the Université catholique de Louvain, Belgium, and the Paris Institute of Political Studies (Sciences Po), France, and is also, since 2020, the United Nations Special Rapporteur on extreme poverty and human rights. He was formerly the United Nations Special Rapporteur on the right to food (from 2008 to 2014) and a member of the United Nations Committee on Economic, Social and Cultural Rights (from 2015 to 2020). A human rights lawyer who specialised in economic and social rights, he previously held various visiting professorships in the United States: at Yale University, at the University of California, Berkeley, and at Columbia University. He was Secretary-General of the International Federation for Human Rights between 2004 and 2008.

Hugh Frazer has worked and written extensively on issues of poverty and social exclusion in Ireland and the EU with a particular focus on child poverty. He is currently Adjunct Professor in Applied Social Studies at Maynooth University, Ireland, and chairperson of Dublin City Community Cooperative, a key community development agency in Dublin's inner city. He is a former Director of the Northern Ireland Voluntary Trust, Northern Ireland's community foundation (1979–1987), and of the Irish government's Combat Poverty Agency (1987–2001). At European level he has worked as an expert on poverty issues in the European Commission (2001–2005) and then as coordinator and social inclusion leader of the European networks of independent experts advising the European Commission on poverty and social Inclusion (2006–2018). He was one of the leading authors of the Feasibility Studies that informed the establishment of the European Child Guarantee.

Anne-Catherine Guio is an economist, with ample expertise in statistics, econometrics and comparative data analysis. She also has a strong interest in qualitative and policy-oriented research. Her main research focuses on material deprivation, poverty, social exclusion and well-being. She has published and lectured extensively in these fields. She is very much involved in research relating to child well-being and child-related policies. She was scientific coordinator of the feasibility study for the European Child Guarantee, and of the follow-up study on the economic implementing framework for this child guarantee. She also coordinated the research that led to the definition of a 'child-specific deprivation indicator', which is now used across the European Union (EU), and in a number of non-EU countries. She is currently Senior Researcher at the Luxembourg Institute of Socio-Economic Research (LISER). Prior to joining LISER, she worked *inter alia* for the EU Statistical Office.

Eric Marlier has been involved, since 1988, in research supported by various international bodies including: the European Commission and other EU institutions, United Nations, OECD and Council of Europe. He manages large-scale research networks such as the EU-funded 'European Social Policy Analysis Network'. He has written and lectured widely on the development of social indicators and their use in the policy process, as well as on comparative social policies and socio-economic data analysis (especially on income and living conditions). He was a member of the World Bank's Commission on Global Poverty, chaired by Sir Tony Atkinson. Through his research and other activities, he is strongly committed to better understanding and improving the situation of children. He is currently International Scientific Coordinator at LISER. Prior to joining LISER, he worked *inter alia* for the Belgian government (private office of the federal Minister for Social Affairs) and the European Commission.

Introduction

Between 1990 and 2015 the number of people in extreme poverty decreased from 1.9 billion to 736 million, and from 36% to 10% of the world's population. The historical decline of poverty continued between 2015 and 2018, with 656 million people in extreme poverty in 2018, and the global poverty rate falling to 8.6%. According to the 2022 Sustainable Development Goals Report (United Nations, 2022), progress would have continued further if it had not been suddenly interrupted by the COVID-19 pandemic and the effects of the war in Ukraine.

Some see this as a success story; but what we need is more humility, not self-congratulation (Alston, 2020). The victory claims noted earlier are conveniently based on the international poverty line used by the World Bank, of US$1.90 per day in 2011 purchasing power parity (PPP). However, although it was raised in November 2022 to US$2.15 per day, this line is so low that even those who do not fall under the threshold may be barely able to survive, let alone live in dignity: in 2020, it corresponded to €1.41 per day in Portugal, to 7.49 yuan per day in China, to 22.49 pesos per day in Mexico, or 355.18 naira per day in Nigeria. No one can seriously contend that one can lead a decent life at or just above such levels of income.

The scorecard is even less impressive once we consider that these global figures on the reduction of poverty have much to do with developments in a single country: China, which has succeeded in reducing poverty from 750 million people in

1990 to 10 million in 2015, and which claims it has succeeded in eradicating extreme poverty entirely since 2021. Moreover, most people who, since the early 1990s, have been raised above the international poverty line, are now just above that line. They are able to escape starvation, thanks to a combination of some income and various solidarity networks. But this cannot plausibly mean that they have overcome poverty.

The failure to eradicate poverty is not only a moral scandal, and an injustice inflicted upon the victim; it also imposes a huge cost on society. In a country such as the United States (US), child poverty costs over US$1 trillion annually, representing 5.4% of its gross domestic product, taking into account the loss of economic productivity, increased health and crime costs, and increased costs as a result of child homelessness and maltreatment. Investing in children, conversely, has considerable returns: for every dollar spent on reducing childhood poverty, seven dollars would be spared (McLaughlin and Rank, 2018).

Why, in a world of plenty, are we failing to eradicate poverty? This collective failure, we believe, is because we only rarely move beyond the symptoms to address the root causes, particularly in early childhood, of the inter-generational perpetuation of poverty (IGPP); because of the efforts of governments being obstructed, in particular as a result of mistaken beliefs concerning 'merit' and 'incentives'; because of the self-interest of and exploitation by some who control excessive wealth and resources; and because of a failure to properly assess the costs to society of poverty and inequalities.

This book argues that we should do more to tackle poverty, and especially that we can do better. Understanding the vicious cycles that perpetuate poverty from one generation to the next is essential to identify which measures can be taken that can break these cycles. While protecting the acquis of the welfare state (where there is one) and strengthening social protection further by a combination of taxation and redistribution are crucial, these efforts will have a limited effect unless we also address the mechanisms that perpetuate poverty: mechanisms that result in children raised in poverty being unable to overcome the disadvantage they encounter in early life.

Equality of opportunity is at the heart of what we propose. Equality of opportunity is often derided as a naïve ideal, or even a conservative objective, both because it is contrasted with equality of outcome and because it is often linked to meritocratic views of society. Taken seriously, however, as a duty of society to address the background conditions that perpetuate poverty, rather than to treat only the symptoms through the classic tools of the welfare state, equality of opportunity can be a radical idea. No child should be penalised for being born in poverty: that idea, which is both simple and, we hope, consensual, can provide the starting point for a much bolder and more imaginative set of policies against poverty.

We are still far today from having realised this ideal of equal opportunity. Children raised in poverty, through no fault of their own, are significantly more likely to remain poor in their adult lives. In a well-publicised report presented in 2018 titled *A Broken Social Elevator?*, the Organisation for Economic Co-operation and Development (OECD) sought to estimate the extent to which the offspring's earnings are related to those of his or her parents. The results are striking: for OECD countries, on average, 40% of the child's earnings in adult life can be attributed to the father's income (OECD, 2018a). Of course, there are important variations between countries, ranging from 10% to 20% (in the Nordic countries) to more than 60% (in Hungary, Luxembourg, Brazil, Colombia and South Africa). But the phenomenon of inter-generational transmission of life chances concerns all countries. Even more important than inheritance of wealth, education and health are the main explanatory factors of this perpetuation of privilege or of disadvantage. Within OECD countries, 63% of children with highly educated parents obtain a college degree, while this is the case for only 15% of children whose parents did not complete secondary school. And the chronic health problems experienced during childhood which result from parents' socioeconomic status, living arrangements and lifestyles significantly increase the probability of poor health in adulthood. This explains why children whose parents are wealthy also have 13% less chances of having a chronic health condition (OECD, 2018a, pp 230–231).

Also in 2018, the World Bank sought to assess the reality of IGPP in different world regions. It found that the inter-generational persistence of privilege at the top quartile of education and of deprivation in the bottom half is far more common than movements up or down (World Bank, 2018, p 125). And what has long been seen as a problem in advanced economies is now even more a problem for the developing world: while individuals born in the 1940s had a higher chance of moving from the bottom half to the top quartile in developing countries than in developed countries, the situation has now reversed – upward mobility is now declining in the developing world, and persistence at the bottom is rising (World Bank, 2018, p 13). As social mobility declines, both privilege and poverty are more likely to persist across generations.

Realising equality of opportunity requires changing the conditions faced by children born in low-income families. And it requires starting at the earliest age, by investing in early childhood education and care: as James Heckman has emphasised, since learning is a cumulative process (the more you have acquired the fundamentals, the better you are equipped to learn further), early interventions are likely to be the most effective in overcoming disadvantage (Heckman, 2006 and 2007).

In this book, we seek to achieve three objectives. Our first objective is to describe the reality of IGPP. We highlight the gap between the ideal of equality of opportunities, on which most societies are built, and the reality of the lives of children born in poverty: we show, in other terms, the various mechanisms that deprive such children of their ability to overcome the circumstances of their birth in their adult lives.

Our second objective, however, is to put will above fate; to pit hope against complacency. The vicious cycles that perpetuate poverty can be broken. The obstacles are neither financial nor lack of knowledge. We now understand much better what should be done, and what is to be done is affordable – especially if we consider the huge costs, at both individual and societal level, of not addressing child poverty more forcefully. What is missing is political will, and perhaps political imagination. We show the political economy obstacles to dealing with child poverty, and we note the paradox that the more affluent a society becomes, the more poverty is mistakenly seen, and described, as a failure of the individual rather than as a failure of society. We also argue that, in order to break the cycles that lead to IGPP, we should move beyond the traditional recipes relying on the stimulation of economic growth, combined with taxes and transfers. Rather than focusing solely or primarily on post-market compensatory measures, our toolkit should put more emphasis on the pre-market mechanisms that cause social exclusion: we outline some elements of what a more inclusive economy could look like.

Our third objective, finally, is to identify some examples of anti-poverty strategies that have worked and thus, with humility, to offer some guidance to policy makers – or at least, to contribute to some form of collective learning. We don't provide a roadmap: not only is the challenge of addressing child poverty enormously complex (and it is certainly not reducible to providing income security to the parents), but in addition solutions that work depend on local contexts and circumstances. What is offered here, then, is rather a set of options, a menu from which to choose, and some general recommendations, such as to ground the anti-poverty strategy in human rights or to ensure meaningful participation of people in poverty, that will be implemented differently depending on specific settings.

The book consists of three main parts. Part I defines the challenge. Chapter One frames the general issue of IGPP.

Chapter Two offers a diagnosis: it seeks to highlight the mechanisms through which poverty is perpetuated from one generation to the next. Part II asks why poverty and inequality matter: Chapter Three presents the case for addressing child poverty as a matter of priority, showing how inaction has corrosive impacts not only for people in poverty themselves, but for society as a whole. Part III turns to solutions. Chapter Four discusses the role of a 'tax-and-transfer' approach to poverty reduction, based on economic growth, combined with progressive taxation and social protection. We argue, however, in Chapter Five that, in addition to this classic approach to poverty reduction, we need to build an inclusive economy: one that prevents exclusion rather than causing exclusion and compensating it *post hoc*. This means, in particular, improving employment opportunities for people in poverty; introducing some form of universal basic income when it matters the most, as young adults enter into their active life; and combating discrimination and stigmatisation. In Chapter Six, finally, we try to address the difficult question of 'how to get there', in other terms, how governments can better equip institutions to meet the challenge of reducing poverty. We examine, for instance, the need for a holistic and integrated approach to the development and delivery of policies to end poverty and social exclusion, or the role of the participation of people in poverty and social exclusion in shaping, implementing and assessing policies aimed at reducing poverty and social exclusion.

PART I

What is IGPP about?

At the outset, it is essential to understand the extent and nature of the challenge we face to ensure the escape from poverty. Thus, we first set out to explain why combating IGPP is key and what the main mechanisms that cause it and perpetuate poverty across generations are. Chapter One defines what the term IGPP means and why it is closely linked to child poverty and to issues of mobility and inequality. Chapter Two then examines the key factors that create vicious cycles that perpetuate poverty across generations. We stress that IGPP is the result of institutional barriers that damage people's development, trap them in poverty and hinder their best efforts to escape. We insist that IGPP is not due to the failings of people living in and growing up in poverty.

ONE

Setting the stage

The inter-generational perpetuation of poverty (IGPP) and its close correlation with child poverty and inequality are the central concerns of this book. Combating child poverty is key to ending IGPP, and ending IGPP, in turn, is essential to reducing child poverty. Likewise, greatly reducing inequality is crucial to ending IGPP and ending IGPP will greatly reduce inequality. The interconnections between these three concepts are introduced in this chapter. We discuss how to define and measure IGPP. We show that children growing up in poverty or social exclusion are more likely to be poor or socially excluded as adults. We look at the evidence of how inequalities have grown, particularly within countries, and assess the efforts to combat (child) poverty and social exclusion. We explain why tackling these is crucial to escaping poverty, and in reviewing the evidence we provide an initial diagnosis of the extent of the challenge.

Defining inter-generational perpetuation of poverty

The shocking and widespread perpetuation of poverty across generations, commonly known as IGPP, occurs when people remain in poverty over a long period and poverty persists from one generation to another. Parents who are poor tend to have children who are poor, who in turn are more likely to become adults who are poor themselves. This perpetuation of poverty across generations is described well by the Chronic Poverty Research Centre (CPRC) as

> the private and public transfer of deficits in assets and resources from one generation to another. Poverty is not transferred inter-generationally as a "package", but as a complex set of positive and negative factors that affect an individual's chances of experiencing poverty in the present or at a future point in their life-course. (Bird and Higgins, 2011, p 9)[1]

Of course, the combination of factors leading to IGPP varies from place to place and family to family. Moreover, there are important structural differences between studying IGPP in developing and Western settings. For example, factors that are normally considered in literature on IGPP in Organisation for Economic Co-operation and Development (OECD) countries include parental endowments and returns on human capital investments. While these remain important in a developing-world context, other factors can be even more important. Examples include lack of access to credit, lack of information, peer and role-model effects and where people

---

[1] In the literature on the perpetuation of poverty, the expression *inter-generational transmission of poverty (IGTP)* is also used to describe this phenomenon. However, this expression can be problematic as the word 'transmission' risks being misinterpreted as 'blaming' parents for the transmission of poverty to their children. This can lead to an overemphasis on personal factors and an insufficient focus on the underlying structural factors that lead to the persistence of poverty from one generation to the next. It risks underplaying the extent to which the persistence of poverty is a symptom of the persistence of deep-seated inequalities from one generation to the next. Thus, we have opted in this book instead for the expression *inter-generational perpetuation of poverty (IGPP)*.

live. The poverty cycle can have more severe consequences in low-income settings, and educational attainment may not necessarily result in occupational mobility. Furthermore, there is a clear difference in data availability, and thus in appropriate methodological approaches, when studying IGPP in a developing-country setting; for example, it is not always helpful to use standardised occupational classifications that were designed to study social mobility in the developed world (Iversen et al, 2019).

Inter-generational perpetuation of poverty and child poverty

IGPP is strongly linked to the widespread persistence of child poverty. Children who grow up in poverty not only have limited opportunities to reach their full potential; they also have a much higher risk of raising their own children in poverty. Household, community and institutional influences affect the development of children's capacities and in due course may result in IGPP, as circumstances in childhood shape later opportunities (Bird and Higgins, 2011).

While IGPP concerns poverty at any age, poverty during childhood can be particularly significant for this process, especially as childhood is such a crucial stage in development (UNICEF and The Global Coalition to End Child Poverty, 2017). The OECD has documented clearly how growing up at the bottom end of the socioeconomic ladder leads to poorer outcomes in almost all well-being areas, and how these well-being inequalities are rooted in the poorer environments that disadvantaged children face at home, in school and in the community (Clarke and Thévenon, 2022). However, while investing in early childhood is critical and cost-effective, it is important to acknowledge that children raised in poverty and deprived of adequate community support are not doomed to fail: essential later treatment and amelioration using evidence-based programmes can also succeed (Rea and Burton, 2019). This means considering the impact of poverty at all stages of childhood, including adolescence, and giving particular attention to transitions (for example, from early childhood education and care [ECEC] to formal schooling, from primary to secondary school and from school to employment). In other words, to counter the dynamic accumulation of disadvantage over the lifecourse it is important to tailor interventions to the appropriate moments and to avoid 'irreversibilities' whenever they may occur.

Children growing up in poverty are more likely to be poor as adults. A study of child poverty in the US, for instance, found that children who experienced poverty at any point during childhood were more than three times as likely to be poor at age 30 as those who were never poor as children. The longer a child was poor, the greater the risk of being poor in adulthood. The incomes of parents and of their children as adults are also closely correlated, especially in developing countries. Perhaps the most striking conclusion from existing studies on IGPP, however, and one we return to later, is that inter-generational mobility decreases as inequality increases: in other terms, in more unequal countries, it is more difficult for children raised in low-income households to overcome this initial disadvantage (UNICEF and The Global Coalition to End Child Poverty, 2017; see also the next section).

These results are confirmed by other studies. In European Union (EU) countries, data on 'intergenerational transmission of disadvantage' collected in 2019 (the most recent available on this topic at the moment of writing this book) confirm that the financial situation of today's adults strongly reflects their living conditions when teenagers. On average in the EU, the at-risk-of-poverty rate was 23.0% among people with a bad financial situation in their household when 14 years old.[2] This

---

[2]   According to the EU definition, a person is 'at risk of poverty' if their equivalent disposable income is below 60% of the national equivalised median income. For the definitions of all EU-agreed indicators, see Social Protection Committee (2022a).

percentage is 9.6 percentage points (pp) higher than the at-risk-of-poverty rate among those with a good financial situation when teenagers (Eurostat, 2021; see also Bellani and Bia, 2017 for an analysis of 2005 and 2011 data on this topic). Similarly, a US study for the National Centre for Children in Poverty in the US shows that poverty rates are much higher among adults who were poor, and especially those highly exposed to poverty, during childhood. For adults who experienced moderate-to-high levels of poverty during childhood (51–100% of childhood years), between 35% and 46% are poor throughout early and middle adulthood (Wagmiller and Adelman, 2009). Thus, combating child poverty is vital to break the vicious cycles that lead poverty to be perpetuated from one generation to the next.

Addressing IGPP is especially urgent today, as the various recent crises have shown that children are particularly vulnerable to shocks. Indeed, the COVID-19 pandemic has led to a significant increase in child poverty: 140 million additional children were living in monetary poor households due to COVID-19, reports UNICEF, and there has been a 14% rise in wasting or malnutrition that may translate into more than 10,000 additional child deaths per month – mostly in sub-Saharan Africa and South Asia (UNICEF, 2020). Many organisations have reported on how COVID-19 has highlighted the impact of pre-existing inequalities on children's physical and mental health and well-being, access to education and continuity of learning, food security and also, in many cases, deepened them further (EU Alliance for Investing in Children, 2020b; Eurochild, 2020; Frazer, 2020; OECD, 2020a and 2020b; Peter G Peterson Foundation, 2021; Yoshida et al, 2020).

Similarly, the current energy and cost-of-living crisis has disproportionally worsened the living conditions of people already poor and increased the number of people falling into poverty. Children are among the most vulnerable in these two groups. According to the United Nations (UN) Development Programme, the soaring food and energy prices have resulted in

71 million people in developing countries falling into poverty (UNDP, 2022).

Without urgent interventions to address the existing and new forms of child poverty resulting from the multiple crises, this is likely to increase the risk of IGPP into the future.

Inter-generational perpetuation of poverty, mobility and inequality

The literature focuses on inter-generational mobility, measured through educational and income mobility, by examining the correlation between parents' and children's income and education (Becker and Tomes, 1986; Mayer and Lopoo, 2005; Mazumder, 2005; Davis and Mazumder, 2022). Relative inter-generational mobility measures the extent to which a person's position in the economic scale (education, income) is independent from his or her parents' position in this scale. Absolute mobility measures the share of people who exceed their parents' standard of living or educational attainment. Both relative and absolute inter-generational mobility is and has been lower in developing countries than in high-income countries (Narayan et al, 2018): while the gap in absolute mobility between high-income and developing countries has been closing, progress in developing economies has stalled since the 1960s and children tend to achieve less educationally than in high-income countries; and developing economies have increasingly fallen behind high-income economies as regards relative inter-generational mobility. Of course, mobility differs across countries. Mobility is lowest in the poorest and most fragile states in the developing world. Educational mobility among low- and middle-income countries varies significantly, being substantially lower in South Asia and sub-Saharan Africa. An OECD study shows that in Nordic countries it would take at least four generations for those born in low-income households to reach the mean income in their society, whereas in emerging countries such as Brazil, Colombia or South Africa, this would take up to nine or even more generations (OECD, 2019a, p 98).

Countries with greater inequality tend to be those where both economic advantage and disadvantage are passed on to children – that is, those in which social mobility is lowest (Corak, 2013; OECD, 2018a; see also Chapter Three). This relationship is often referred to as the 'Great Gatsby Curve'. The name was initially proposed by Alan Krueger, a former head of the Council of Economic Advisors to the President of the US, referring to F. Scott Fitzgerald's novel *The Great Gatsby*. But it is a strange choice, when you think of it: in the novel, the eponymous character, Jay Gatsby, embodies the concept of mobility, rising from being a bootlegger to leading the Long Island north shore social set; yet, what the 'Great Gatsby Curve' shows is that this kind of rise is the exception rather than the rule, and that it is especially unlikely in highly unequal societies.

The lesson from the 'Great Gatsby Curve' is clear: unless we tackle wealth and income inequality more seriously, we will be unable to ensure social mobility. In other terms, true equality of opportunities requires that we do more to ensure that we reduce disparities in children's access to resources. As quipped by the dean of studies on inequality, Tony Atkinson: 'Inequality of outcome among today's generation is the source of the unfair advantage received by the next generation. If we are concerned about equality of opportunity tomorrow, we need to be concerned about inequality of outcome today' (Atkinson, 2015).

Considerable effort is still required in this area. Since 1980, half of the world's income has been in the hands of the top 10%. The income share of the top 1% has in fact kept increasing, from 16% in 1980 to 19% in 2021, while the share of the global bottom 50% stagnated between 6% and 9%.[3] The speed at

---

[3]   Pre-tax income estimates of population over 20. World Inequality Database, https://wid.world/share/#0/countriestimeseries/sptinc_p9 0p100_z/WO;QB;QD;XL;QE/last/eu/k/p/yearly/s/false/28.9715/ 70/curve/false/country

which incomes are growing is also unequal: in three-quarters of OECD countries, incomes of households of the top 10% have grown faster than those of the poorest 10% (Cingano, 2014, para 7). Income distribution is also unequal within specific regions/countries. The world's three most unequal regions are Latin America, the Middle East and North Africa (MENA) and the sub-Saharan region, where the top 10% earned around 55% of the national income (World Inequality Database, accessed in March 2023). These are followed closely by Asia (where this share is 50%). The evolution of inequality may also differ. Whereas the share earned by the top 10% in Asian countries decreased slightly between 1980 and 2021 (from 54.4% to 50.3%), in Europe it *increased* (from 31.2% to 36.2%). In Russia, the share of the top 10% increased from 22% in 1980 to 51% in 2021 and the share of the top 1% from 4% to 24%. The corresponding figures for China and India regarding the evolution of the top 1% are respectively 7% to 16% and 8% to 22% (World Inequality Database, accessed in March 2023).

Wealth inequality is even greater, and has grown even faster, than income inequality. Across the OECD, the wealthiest 10% hold 52% of total net wealth. In turn, the 60% least wealthy households own a little over 12% of total wealth, and over a third of people with incomes above the poverty line in the OECD lack the financial resources necessary to deal with sudden loss of income, for instance in case of unemployment, family breakdown or illness (Balestra and Tonkin, 2018, para 6). In the US in 2019, one third of households with children were net-worth poor (assets less total debts below the federal poverty line), three times as many as those who were income poor (Gibson-Davis et al, 2021).

Economic poverty can be transmitted through the transmittance of debt, inheritance practices and lack of assets. This is true in both developing and rich countries, and it is why it is important to address wealth inequalities in addition to income inequalities (OECD, 2018b). Losing assets can lead to downward mobility, and lack of assets can be associated with poverty traps, showing that deficits in assets are important in driving IGPP (Bird and Higgins, 2011). Deficit of assets such as not owning land will have an impact on an offspring's life chances. Households living with insufficient resources are also less able to deal with external shocks, such as a household member dying, environmental disasters causing displacement, or conflict, and this can further trap them in poverty and often result in downward mobility. Such emergencies, economic and humanitarian crises disproportionately affect the poorest.

TWO

How poverty is perpetuated across generations

The factors that lead to the perpetuation of poverty from one generation to the next are many. They include not only lack of sufficient income but also limited access to essential services such as education, healthcare and nutrition, poor housing conditions and poor employment prospects. Fewer opportunities for saving, acquiring or inheriting assets, and low coverage by social protection mechanisms mean that people experiencing poverty rarely have a chance to change their trajectories. While richer households respond to external and internal shocks with their accumulated wealth and earnings, social networks and higher education levels that enable them to get better-paid jobs, poorer individuals have fewer options to mitigate risks and shocks. Poor access to healthcare and exposure to risk factors can lead to poor health. Poor health is not only costly where health insurance is insufficient or unavailable; it also reduces employment opportunities. Living in substandard housing conditions or in locations underserved by public services may also have significant impacts on the ability to escape poverty. Access to quality education, including early childhood education, is also often more difficult for families on low incomes, and educational achievement is significantly impeded by circumstances faced in early childhood. Access to sport, culture and leisure activities are also often limited, thus curtailing development opportunities. Employment prospects are also weaker, for reasons linked to socioeconomic disadvantage during childhood. Discrimination and intra-household dynamics, including the impacts of poverty-related stress on the child's early development and on gender inequality (as women disproportionately shoulder the burden of a lack of access to essential services), also play important roles in perpetuating poverty. In addition, environmental shocks and climate change are increasingly important factors. Evidence also suggests that violent conflict causes and intensifies poverty and its persistence (Rohwerder, 2014).

Key factors causing and perpetuating IGPP:

- Growing up on an insufficient income and lack of adequate social protection
- Poor health and poor access to health services
- Malnutrition
- Living in inadequate housing and in disadvantaged neighbourhoods
- Insufficient access to early childhood care and education
- Experiencing educational disadvantage and poor access to good-quality primary and secondary education
- Limited access to sport, culture and leisure activities
- Poor access to decent employment
- Discrimination, stereotyping and prejudice
- Gender inequality and intra-household dynamics
- Environmental shocks and climate change
- Poverty-related stress and the undermining of people's aspirations, self-confidence and hope
- Violent conflict and population displacement

These various factors are examined later in the chapter. Often, they work in combination, reinforcing one another, creating the conditions for systemic forms of exclusion. For instance, poor health combined with low levels of education will result in diminished employment opportunities, which in turn will lead to insufficient investment in preventative healthcare and in education, thus perpetuating poverty. Low-income households live in disadvantaged neighbourhoods, because housing is unaffordable elsewhere: as a result, children typically attend lower-quality schools, and the adults can only find employment in places distant from their homes – with long commuting times making it more difficult for them to support the children in their homework or even to serve them home-cooked, nourishing meals. And so forth.

Health

Just as poverty results in poor health outcomes, ill health imposes a burden on households that may worsen their economic insecurity and lead to catastrophic expenditures, higher debt levels and the selling of productive assets. This is the vicious cycle between poverty and health.

Poverty, inequality and ill health

Poverty and ill health are interrelated. Disadvantaged groups are more often exposed to a large range of risks to health, including environmental hazards or extreme temperatures, and to financial barriers in accessing healthcare. The increased exposure to poverty-related risk factors results in major differences in life expectancy between poor people and the rest of the population. According to one study in the US, individuals living in poverty have 10.5 years' lower life expectancy than middle-income earners (Singh and Lee, 2021). This confirms findings from earlier studies in the US, including one study showing that the richest 1% of women and men live respectively 10.1 and 14.6 years longer on average than the poorest 1%, and that life expectancy over the period 2001–14 grew twice as fast for those in the top 5% as for those in the bottom 5% (Chetty et al, 2016).

Poverty kills. The situation of the US is not unique: across EU countries, 30-year-old men with less than upper secondary education can expect to live about eight years less than those with a tertiary education, on average (OECD and European Union, 2018, p 84). In England, the difference in life expectancy between the richest and the poorest was 9.3 years for men and 7.3 for women in 2018 (Public Health England, 2018, ch 5), and between 2003 and 2018, one in three premature deaths was attributable to neighbourhood deprivation: if everyone had the same risk of mortality as those in high-income brackets, almost 900,000 premature deaths would have been prevented throughout this period (Lewer et al, 2020).

In turn, poor health leads to poverty, both because of the reduced productivity of workers and due to the costs of seeking healthcare. At least half of the world's population cannot get the healthcare it needs. In 2010, an estimated 808 million people spent more than 10% of their household's total consumption or income on out-of-pocket health expenses, and almost 100 million people (97% of them in Africa and Asia) are pushed into extreme poverty each year because of out-of-pocket health expenses (World Health Organization and International Bank for Reconstruction and Development [WHO and IBRD]/ The World Bank, 2017, p 24). Nearly half of Africans did not seek needed healthcare in 2014–15, and four in ten of those who did had difficulty in accessing that care (Afrobarometer, 2017, p 7).

In addition to direct financial barriers such as user fees, insufficient access to healthcare is explained in certain countries by the fear of discrimination or stigmatisation, lack of education and transportation, and corruption (Hsiao et al, 2019): one in seven (14%) of those who accessed health services on the African continent has paid a bribe to obtain them (Afrobarometer, 2017, p 7). Informal payments or bribery not only lead to high out-of-pocket spending on health: they also erode public trust in the healthcare system, and lead to reduced service utilisation (Naher et al, 2020). An estimated 10–25% of the US$7 trillion world health spending is lost to corruption; this is more than the amount needed each year to ensure universal healthcare globally by 2030, according to WHO estimates (García, 2019).

As well as poverty, inequality is a key factor in poor health. More equal societies have healthier populations: the correlation between greater income equality and improved health outcomes (measured by indicators such as life expectancy or infant mortality) holds for both developed and developing countries (Babones, 2008; Pickett and Wilkinson, 2015). In Africa and Latin America, health outcomes – including life expectancy – were significantly worsened by the growth of inequalities; increases in gross domestic product (GDP) per capita do not make up for this (Odusanya and Akinio, 2021; Biggs et al, 2010). Evidence from these regions shows that GDP growth does not automatically lead to better health; how this increased prosperity is redistributed matters far more than the average increase itself.

Poverty and children's health

The health impacts of growing up in poverty are particularly severe on children. Poorer children often have worse health than other children and find it more difficult to access health services. The stress from living in scarcity leads to a physiological response: increased levels of stress hormones, the most well-known of which are the corticotropin-releasing hormone, cortisol, norepinephrine and adrenaline – which, while a natural and to a certain extent protective body reaction, may damage the brain if prolonged at high levels (Reynolds, 2013; Barboza Solís et al, 2015). Stress can also damage the functioning of the prefrontal cortex, and thus impair learning, the regulation of behaviour and interpersonal relationships (Hanson et al, 2013). A committee of the American Academy of Paediatrics summarised this evidence by noting that 'poverty and other social determinants of health adversely affect relational health', which, 'particularly in the absence of emotional support by a nurturing adult, increases the risk of childhood toxic stress and difficulties in emotional regulation, early child development, and eventually, lifelong health' (Pascoe et al, 2016).

According to UNICEF, 22,000 children die each day due to poverty, mostly from preventable conditions and diseases (UNICEF and the Global Coalition to End Child Poverty, 2017). Early childhood is a major driver of inequalities in health. As EuroHealthNet has pointed out, this is because adversity at this early stage of life tends to have a negative effect on all the different domains of child development – cognitive, communication and language, social and emotional skills. Inadequate development of these skills has a profound effect on outcomes across the remainder of the lifecourse (Goldblatt et al, 2015).

A key dimension of growing up in economic poverty is the negative impact on mental health of the daily struggle to survive. Using data collected in the third wave of Children's Worlds, the school-based survey of children in 35 countries, Gross-Manos and Bradshaw (2022) have highlighted that at the macro-country level, material deprivation and multidimensional poverty showed high correlations with overall life satisfaction and feelings of sadness of children. Suffering includes negative thoughts and emotions, including stress, fear, anxiety and shame (Bray et al, 2019). Children in particular deal with stress and are affected by their parents' stress (Khan et al, 2020). This undermining of mental health and feeling of stress can have an especially negative effect on children and influence IGPP, as it can impact on cognitive functioning and emotional well-being, and there is evidence of a biological transmission of stress (Bowers and Yehuda, 2016). Evidence shows that when babies and children experience strong, frequent and/or extended periods of stress due to social conditions such as poverty or even abusive treatment or mental illness, they can experience toxic stress, which has long-term consequences for learning, behaviour and both physical and mental health. This in turn will likely have consequences for later educational and occupational attainment (McEwen and McEwen, 2017).

While the risk of poor health is greatly increased by growing up on an inadequate income and a range of other social determinants, this is often compounded by poor children having poorer access to essential health services.

This is particularly true in countries with public healthcare of low quality, insufficient coverage and high out-of-pocket payments. However, even in the regions of the world with developed and accessible healthcare services and low unmet medical need for children in general, poor and non-poor children still have differential access to healthcare. In Europe, the latest data on children's unmet need for healthcare (collected in 2021) show that while the percentage of children with unmet need is quite low, with an average of 2.8% for medical care and 3.6% for dental care, those living in poverty suffer from two times more unmet need for medical care or unmet need for dental care than non-poor children (EU Statistics on Income and Living Conditions [EU-SILC] Users' Data Base 2021, authors' calculations). However, these differences are not present in all EU Member States – showing that there is no inevitability in this gap.

Data on other parts of the world are scarce but confirm such differences, with specific contextual difficulties. For instance, in South Africa the major social determinants of bad health in children are poverty, food insecurity, inadequate housing and living in rural areas, where the majority of children experiencing poverty reside (Alternate Report Coalition – Children's Rights South Africa [ARC-CRSA], 2016). The difference in health between rural and urban areas is striking: approximately twice the proportion of rural children are affected by health deprivation in comparison to urban areas. This is largely due to long distances which must be travelled to healthcare services in rural areas, the quality of those services and bad housing conditions (Maluleke, 2020).

Impact of poverty on children's future health prospects and IGPP

Conditions in childhood determine health outcomes later in life. The benefits of healthy childhood development extend to older ages, as highlighted in evidence from longitudinal studies: birth weight, infant growth and peak physical and cognitive capacities in childhood are associated with or predictive of older adults' physical and cognitive capacities, muscle strength, bone mass, lens opacity, hearing capacity, skin thickness and life expectancy (The Lancet, 2020). Adults with an early experience of poverty during childhood are at a higher risk of developing hypertension, chronic inflammation or immune-mediated chronic diseases (Miller et al, 2011; Ziol-Guest et al, 2012). In developing countries, stunting and wasting are often serious issues resulting from inadequate nutrition during childhood (see next section). These have dire consequences for IGPP, as the negative effects of poor health in childhood resulting from growing up in poverty can cause long-term damage to people's health later in life and lead to lower productivity and earnings over a lifetime.

In conclusion, poverty affects both the long-term health prospects of individuals and their economic prospects because of its impacts on the child's development. The health effects of child poverty seem to be one of the major factors in IGPP.

Nutrition

Households living on low incomes will generally seek to cut down on food expenses, which is often the first item that is sacrificed in times of crisis: they shift to less diversified diets, they reduce the portions or they skip meals. Poverty thus results in malnutrition, whether in the form of undernutrition (which translates into wasting, stunting or being underweight), of micronutrient deficiency due to a lack of vitamins or minerals, or of unbalanced diets leading to overweight and obesity.

This in turn exposes household members to diet-related non-communicable diseases, such as type 2 diabetes or heart diseases, thus increasing healthcare costs, reducing productivity and slowing economic growth. This, a report of the WHO notes, 'can perpetuate a cycle of poverty and ill-health' (WHO, 2021). Today, 821 million people globally face food insecurity, to a large extent as a result of being poor; 1.9 billion adults are overweight or obese, while 462 million are underweight.

Impact of poverty on child nutrition

Growing up with insufficient resources often leads to inadequate nutrition or malnutrition. In 2020, 149 million children across the world under the age of five were estimated to be stunted (too short for their age), 45 million were estimated to be wasted (too thin for their height) and 38.9 million were overweight or obese. Around 45% of deaths among children under five years of age are linked to undernutrition, mostly in low- and middle-income countries. At the same time, in these same countries, rates of childhood overweight and obesity are rising. These countries thus face a 'triple burden': undernutrition and micronutrient deficiency persist, while obesity is emerging as a new and major public health challenge (WHO, 2021).

In high-income countries, low-income households tend to shift to poorly diversified diets and low-cost food options, including energy-dense foods that require little or no preparation, since cooking meals requires time and raises energy bills. Child nutrition is obviously affected. In EU countries for instance, according to the latest data available (2021), children in poverty have five times more risk to lack proteins or fresh fruits and vegetables daily. It is only in most Nordic countries, Cyprus and Luxembourg that differences are negligible (EU-SILC Users' Data Base 2021, authors' calculations). These data underline the importance of ensuring that children, and in particular poor children, have access to free full meals at school (Guio, 2023).

Lack of income is not the only factor. Other key factors increase the risks of malnutrition among children growing up in poverty. These include: the time-poverty affecting low-income families; the physical food environments, including 'food deserts' (where access to fresh and healthy food items is difficult) and 'food swamps' (where local food outlets primarily sell processed and unhealthy food options); the lack of, or inadequate or unaffordable, meals in schools, ECEC centres and other public services and the lack of such provision during school holidays; a lack of awareness of what constitutes a healthy diet and food supply; marketing that promotes unhealthy foods; and insufficient policies and programmes to promote mother and child health, in particular breastfeeding (Bradshaw and Rees, 2019; Frazer et al, 2020). Social norms – how people eat – also have an impact: studies show, for instance, that when people eat as a 'secondary activity' (in other terms, when they eat while watching television or while studying, and so forth), they consume more calories per time unit; and the time-poverty many low-income households face, linked in part to the long commuting times between home and work, may result in fewer meals being taken together, and more meals being taken 'on the move', while doing something else (Bertrand and Whitmore Schanzenback, 2009).

Of course, in conflict-ridden regions, such conflicts and humanitarian crises are also key factors in increasing malnutrition, as they greatly increase the level of food insecurity. According to the Global Report on Food Crises (World Food Programme, 2022), in 2021, around 139 million people were facing food crises across 24 countries/territories where conflict/insecurity was considered the primary driver. The report also shows that the impact of weather-related disasters (in the form of drought, rainfall deficits, flooding and cyclones) has been particularly detrimental in key crises in East, Central and Southern Africa, in 2021. Food price inflation is another key driver of food insecurity, which increased during the post-pandemic period and has been further exacerbated by the Ukraine conflict.

Impact of childhood malnutrition on children's future prospects and IGPP

The connection between low income and inadequate nutrition has serious consequences, as adequate child nutrition is critical to healthy development, particularly at birth and during infancy: this is often described as the 'first 1,000 days-window', to refer to the time between the start of pregnancy and the second birthday of the child as the key period during which nutrition will play a major role in the child's physical and intellectual development. Adequate nutrition helps to achieve or maintain not only a normal body weight and height, according to age, gender and race, but also a good state of physical and mental health. It consists of a balanced diet, based on the consumption of a variety of foods, containing adequate proportions of carbohydrates, fats and proteins, along with the recommended daily allowances of all essential minerals and vitamins (Food and Agriculture Organization [FAO] and WHO, 2019). If school-age children are hungry they will not learn successfully, which has an impact on their future prospects as adults; moreover, poor health or obesity resulting from inadequate nutrition during early childhood will reduce productivity at work and expose to discrimination, thus affecting access to employment (Bradshaw and Rees, 2019; Drèze, 2019; Frazer et al, 2020). A WHO study in 2013–14 provided information on, among other things, the prevalence of overweight and obesity among girls and boys aged 11 in 42 countries and regions across Europe and North America: in about half of the countries covered, low family income was linked to overweight and obesity for boys, and this was true for girls in two-thirds of the countries (Inchley et al, 2016). As well as the importance of early years, UNICEF and WHO have also focused on the nutrition, health and well-being of adolescent girls, as mothers-to-be, recognising that maternal under-nutrition impacts infants' birth weight, and may affect growth and development, perpetuating an inter-generational vicious cycle (Dornan and Woodhead, 2015). Finally, food habits during childhood also have long-term consequences on healthy food habits as adults and parents.

Housing and living environment

People who are poor don't choose where they live: they opt for neighbourhoods where rent is affordable. As a result, however, they may be far from employment opportunities, live in heavily polluted or toxic environments, with fewer green areas and thus incentives to exercise outdoors, and with lower-quality public services. They also often live in dwellings that are too small, poorly insulated or otherwise inadequate. This has a long-term impact on people's chances of escaping poverty (Bartlett, 1998; Tunstall et al, 2013). More than 1.8 billion people worldwide lack adequate housing, and at least 1 billion people live in informal settlements (Farha, 2020). Homelessness, the most severe violation of the right to adequate housing, affects about 150 million people globally (United Nations Economic and Social Council, 2020). People living in poverty obviously have a higher risk of worse housing conditions than others; this in turn imposes on them further disadvantages, creating the conditions for the perpetuation of poverty.

Impact of poverty on access to decent housing and safe living environment

Children's health and well-being depend to a large extent on whether they have access to adequate housing and can live in safe environments; these conditions also are a major determinant of their ability to perform well at school. In the EU, the 2013 EU Recommendation on Investing in Children acknowledges the importance of safe and adequate housing and of a child-friendly living environment. The recommendation encourages EU Member States to ensure households with children can live in affordable quality housing; to reduce exposure to environmental hazards, overcrowding and energy poverty; to support households and children at risk of homelessness; to pay attention to children's best interests in local planning and avoid 'ghettoisation' and segregation; and to reduce children's harmful exposure to a deteriorating living and social environment to prevent them from falling victim to violence and abuse (European Commission, 2013). More recently, the 2021 European Child Guarantee highlights the need to ensure that 'children in need' have effective access to adequate housing (Council of the EU, 2021).

Substandard housing

Children from socioeconomically disadvantaged households are more likely to grow up in overcrowded, poorly insulated housing, exposed to polluted and unsafe environments. They are also more likely to live in neighbourhoods that are ghettoised, violent and with inadequate access to essential services, as we further discuss later. These living conditions affect health, of course, both because of housing conditions as such – including exposure to high levels of air pollution, especially where clean energy is inaccessible or regulation is insufficient (Scott, 2006) – and because of poor food environments[1] and limited access to green areas for physical exercise and leisure (Kawachi and Berkman, 2003). Overcrowded living conditions may lead to disturbed sleep, tenser family relationships and stress and anxiety, negatively affecting children's education and causing depression (Reynolds and Robinson, 2005).

Poor neighbourhoods

The quality of neighbourhoods has a significant impact on social mobility. Children growing up in areas in which poverty

---

[1] Food environments refers to 'the physical, economic, political and socio-cultural context in which consumers engage with the food system to make their decisions about acquiring, preparing, and consuming food' (High Level Panel of Experts on Food Security and Nutrition [HLPE], 2017, p 28). As already noted, in low-income neighbourhoods, access to healthy food options may be difficult, as such neighbourhoods may be 'food deserts' or 'food swamps'.

is concentrated, such as decaying areas of industrial cities or isolated rural communities, are likely to have poorer access to services and facilities and may be more at risk of violence and abuse, as shown by studies in the EU (Eurochild and European Anti-Poverty Network [EAPN], 2013). The American Academy of Paediatrics has noted that poor neighbourhoods expose families to a variety of barriers and harms, and low-income areas also may lack quality schools, sustainable jobs, healthcare facilities, safe recreation spaces and other resources that support healthy community activities (Pascoe et al, 2016). Children growing up in deprived communities also often lack access to green spaces. For instance, a study in Dublin has shown that the inner city has significantly less green open spaces than other parts of Dublin (Kelly, 2016); and the impacts are compounded by the fact that many families live in small flats, apartments or houses with no gardens. Thus, the historic physical neglect of more disadvantaged communities in Dublin in terms of the provision of quality outdoor space for recreational use has fundamentally exacerbated the stress and tension of an already difficult situation for these communities and families (Frazer, 2020). This is important, given the growing body of literature on 'nature deficit disorder' (Louv, 2009; Richardson and Hallam, 2013) and the contribution that a relationship with nature can play in reducing Attention Deficit Hyperactivity Disorder (Amoly et al, 2014).

Impact of housing conditions and living environment during childhood on children's future prospects and IGPP

Children raised in substandard housing and poor areas experience multiple disadvantages, resulting in these children and their families being trapped in poverty and unable to escape. Housing conditions affect social relationships and life chances generally (van Ham et al, 2014). Poor housing conditions (such as lack of light or space to play), the American Academy of Paediatrics has warned, cause ill-health or accidents; and result in lower educational outcomes and reduced general well-being as well as in an increased risk of perpetuating the inter-generational poverty cycle (with profound and long-term effects on children's life chances) (Pascoe et al, 2016).

Housing conditions per se are not the only issue; the quality of neighbourhoods plays an equally important role. Poor and segregated neighbourhoods mean children will have fewer social connections and less quality schools. As young adults, they will lack decent job opportunities. And access to proper healthcare services may be more difficult, resulting in a reduced reliance on preventive healthcare. Residential segregation thus reduces equality of opportunities.

There is an emerging body of literature on IGPP on what is known as the 'neighbourhood effect' in Western countries (de Vuijst et al, 2017), which provides growing evidence that not just parent-to-child interactions but also neighbourhood interactions can influence IGPP. Generally, researchers have identified four factors in this effect, including: isolation from supportive social networks; loss of mutual trust and control over youth behaviour; inadequate public and school resources; and harm from environmental hazards (McEwen and McEwen, 2017). Research in the US has shown that inter-generational mobility varies substantially across areas within the US. Chetty et al estimate the likelihood that a child from a household in the bottom quintile of the (national) income distribution will make it into the top quintile: this likelihood varies by a factor of about 2.8 across the country (from about one in 25 in Charlotte, NC to around one in eight in San Jose, Silicon Valley). The factors correlated with upward mobility are: (i) less residential segregation; (ii) less income inequality; (iii) better primary schools; (iv) greater social capital; and (v) greater family stability (Chetty et al, 2014). An experiment held in the US offered randomly selected families housing vouchers to move from high-poverty areas to better-off neighbourhoods. The results illustrate the potentially powerful impacts of residential desegregation on social mobility: in the households that moved to better-off areas, long-term college attendance and earnings in adult life for children increased, especially for children who were exposed to better-off neighbourhoods before the age of 13 (Chetty et al, 2016).

There is less research on the neighbourhood effect and its part in IGPP in developing countries. It is likely, however, that the effect is even more pronounced in these countries, as there are larger within-country differences in public goods, quality of schools and marginalisation of groups (Iversen et al, 2019). As in the US, research in Africa (Alesina et al, 2019) and India (Asher et al, 2021) on inter-generational mobility points to stark variations across locations, and often within small areas (such as the Delhi neighbourhoods). In India, upward mobility is higher in areas that are southern, urban, with high average education levels and manufacturing employment. Access to community networks, to peer groups and role models, and to quality healthcare and education services also play an important role in developing countries, which further underlines the importance of combating residential segregation (Munshi, 2011; Iversen et al, 2019).

Education

Access to education, both primary and secondary and also early childhood, is often seen as one of the key routes out of poverty. Yet, children raised in poverty benefit less from education than their peers, and at times education systems can contribute to perpetuating poverty and inequality. As a result, adults living in poverty often cannot ensure means for their children to grow up with better opportunities than they had, despite their best efforts to do so. Many parents express the hope that their children will go to school and even complete a university education (World Bank, 2018, p 117). Yet, being raised in a disadvantaged family has significant impacts on access to education and on educational achievement.

Impact of poverty on early childhood education and care

Improving ECEC is essential to break the cycles of poverty, because it is during this time period that the impacts of poverty on the child's future prospects are most significant. Interventions in early-age childhood are particularly effective at closing the gap between disadvantaged children and their wealthier peers, as compared with later-life remediation efforts (Heckman and Mosso, 2014). (Affordable and easily accessible childcare facilities also present another advantage: they significantly raise women's employment prospects, and thus the ability for households to improve their standards of living and, in turn, to invest in education.) At the same time, it is important to avoid any sense of fate: while the stress of poverty on the family may have severe impacts on the child (including on the child's brain development), these impacts are not inevitable, and they can be reversed: programmes supporting parental engagement and relational health can effectively buffer the chronic stress of poverty (Larson et al, 2015). Parenting during the early years plays a crucial role, and it should not be affected by socioeconomic disadvantage: this is why support to parents should be treated as a priority.

Indeed, reading books to children and having conversations with them is a major determinant of the acquisition of verbal skills (Rowe, 2017), and a critical source of stimulation for child development (Heckman, 2006) But poverty-related concerns consume mental resources, leaving less for other tasks (Mani et al, 2013), such as meaningfully interacting with children. Language-rich interactions between parents and children are in turn more common in affluent families, because of the time constraints parents face in low-income families and in single-parent families in particular; because of the generally lower education levels of low-income parents; and because of the stress associated with economic insecurity, which often reduces the availability of parents for such interactions (OECD, 2019b). For example, in Paraguay, 90% of children in the richest 20%

of households benefit from stimulating adult engagement, but only 40% of children in the poorest 20% do so (United Nations Educational, Scientific and Cultural Organization [UNESCO], 2020, p 232). In the US, children from professional families have been found to speak more than twice as many words as children from families in poverty (Heckman and Mosso, 2014, p 8). These children have also benefited from exposure to a larger set of formative experiences: between birth and age six, low-income children in the US spend nearly 1,300 fewer hours in novel places and 400 fewer hours on literacy activities than high-income children (Phillips, 2011, pp 217, 221).

Impact of poverty on primary and secondary education achievements

Save the Children provides an apt summary of the link between poverty and educational disadvantage: 'Poverty has an impact on children's educational achievements. It impairs their performance at school, hinders development of their talents and limits their aspirations. Child poverty not only affects early childhood, it also jeopardises children's futures' (Save the Children, 2016). Across the EU-27, there is a strong link between experiencing poverty in childhood and inequality in educational attainment. Research shows that only '19% of those who had experienced "bad" or "very bad" financial circumstances in childhood had attained a tertiary education in adulthood, compared to 43.7% of those whose childhood circumstances had been "good" or "very good"' (Curristan et al, 2022). In the light of this, one would hope that schools would be institutions compensating for inequalities between children of different socioeconomic backgrounds. Instead, schools tend to reproduce such hierarchies, at worst magnifying them further. Four specific mechanisms are at work.

First, children from disadvantaged backgrounds may face obstacles in their access to quality education. In low- and lower-middle-income countries, the likelihood of enrolment in primary, lower-secondary and upper-secondary school still depends on parental income and education levels to a significant extent (World Bank, 2018, p 120). Officially, education is provided free of charge almost universally. But extra fees related to school supplies and learning materials, as well as transportation, still prevent children from disadvantaged families from access to schools. In contrast, high-income families can spend money, not only on school fees, but also on additional expenditure including computers, high-quality childcare, summer camps, private schooling and other things that promote the capacities of their children. In the US, for example, the additional school expenditure of families in the top 20% more than doubled between the early 1970s and early 2000s, while that of families in the bottom 20% remained virtually static and was seven times lower in the mid-2000s (Duncan and Murnane, 2011).

Second, children from poor families can also suffer marginalisation in school, due to their social origin. For example, one in ten children in European OECD countries lacks access to basic clothing (OECD, 2019b, p 60), which can lead those children to be discriminated against, excluded or bullied at school both by their peers and by school staff. A participatory action research project on education in Belgium identified that shame experienced by children in poverty was one of the key obstacles to successful schooling (ATD Quart Monde and Changement pour l'Egalité, 2017, p 12). There may be stigmatisation, labelling and negative assumptions about children in poverty.

Third, children from higher socioeconomic backgrounds tend to be better prepared for formal education, in terms of both cognitive abilities and social behaviour. Where children from poor families exhibit learning deficiencies, these often appear even before they are enrolled in school. As a result, across nearly all countries, the family background of a student (parental education, socioeconomic status, conditions at home) remains the single most important predictor of learning outcomes: the OECD's Programme for International Student

Assessment (PISA) tests, which are taken every three years, indicated in 2018 that pupils aged 15 from less privileged social backgrounds performed less well at school than their better-off peers. Some of the most marginalised groups, such as Roma children and children from a migrant background and who experience a culmination of disadvantages (for example, extreme deprivation, cultural and language barriers and discrimination), have particularly low educational outcomes (Frazer et al, 2020).

While assessments of academic achievements are often biased against children from low socioeconomic backgrounds (UNESCO, 2020, p 221), the gaps in educational outcomes between children from wealthy and poor families remain constant as children grow (Ermisch et al, 2012, pp 465, 468). One reason behind this unfair gap is that time spent at school brings fewer benefits for children from low-income families than for their better-off peers (OECD, 2015a, p 27), a phenomenon significantly worsened by low-quality teaching. Globally, 125 million children are not literate or numerate after spending four years in school, with the largest deficits incurred by children in poverty (World Bank, 2018, p 78). In seven sub-Saharan African countries, students were found to receive just under three hours of teaching per day, or half of the scheduled time, and large shares of teachers were not properly trained in their teaching area (Bold et al, 2017).

Indeed, the quality – or perceived quality – of schooling can also discourage children and parents from formal education. The belief that school is a waste of time and/or money weighs in the trade-off between sending children to school or to work. Given the constraints they face and the high opportunity costs when children could be working to sustain their families, poor parents who perceive education to be of low quality may be less willing to keep their children in school (Bold et al, 2017). Child labour can then be an important reason for poor school performance and school dropout. About one in ten children aged 5 to 17 years were engaged in child labour worldwide in 2016 (International Labour Organization and the United Nations Children's Fund [ILO and UNICEF], 2021). Of these, one third do not attend school at all; the others go to school, but not all the time. Children in child labour are more likely to leave school early, before grade completion, and underperform in tests (Thévenon and Edwards, 2019). Enforcing laws and regulations prohibiting child labour and strengthening child protection systems can play a crucial role in reducing levels of child labour (Thévenon and Edwards, 2019). Although child labour fell by 94 million between 2000 and 2016, it has continued rising since, reaching a total of 160 million and with a sharp increase due to the COVID-19 pandemic (ILO and UNICEF, 2021).

Finally, the level of education of parents has a significant impact on the benefits children may obtain from education. For instance, one study highlighted that in countries such as France, Japan, South Korea and the United Kingdom (UK), the offspring of parents from low-education groups earned 20% less than their peers with parents from high-education groups, even with the same level of qualifications (Jerrim and Macmillan, 2015). This may act as a strong disincentive to invest in education: why would one put efforts into performing well at school, if this will not be rewarded in the world of work?

The educational achievement of children thus depends on the socioeconomic status of their parents. Even more troubling, the gap between those at the top and the bottom is increasing. A study analysing 100 countries and about 5.8 million students found that the gap increased between 1964 and 2015 based on parent occupation (with an increase of 55%), parent education (50%), as well as the presence of books in the household (40%): students' family's socioeconomic status and cultural capital (for which the presence of books is a strong indicator) play an increasingly decisive role. Moreover, the gaps have increased more between the middle and bottom of the income distribution than between the middle and the top: the academic opportunities of children of low-income families have particularly decreased (Chmielewski, 2019).

In some countries, conflict situations worsen educational disadvantage. Research on Africa points to substantive educational mobility setbacks in countries either vulnerable to or experiencing conflict (Alesina et al, 2019). On the other hand, education makes people resilient to shocks such as conflict, and it is a 'portable' asset of great value (Bird et al, 2010).

Impact of education on children's future prospects and IGPP

Highlighting the critical role that preschool and school can play in breaking IGPP, UNICEF writes that 'without quality education, disadvantaged children are far more likely to be trapped as adults in low-skilled, poorly paid and insecure employment, preventing them from breaking inter-generational cycles of disadvantage' (UNICEF, 2016; also Dornan and Woodhead, 2015). Curristan et al (2022) show that in Ireland, educational attainment explains 10pp of the difference in adult deprivation outcomes between those who experienced 'very bad' childhood circumstances and those who experienced 'very good' childhood circumstances.

One of the keys to breaking the cycle of poverty is ensuring that children growing up in poverty have access to high-quality inclusive education that enables them to reach their full potential and to positively influence aspirations and attitudes. These returns on investment are particularly important in low-income and lower-middle-income countries. UNICEF estimates that 'On *average*, each additional year of education a child receives increases her or his adult earnings by about 10%. And for each additional year of schooling completed, on average, by young adults in a country, that country's poverty rate falls by 9%' (UNICEF, 2016). Education for girls is particularly important in breaking the cycle of poverty, as education empowers girls later in life to seek better healthcare during pregnancy, in childbirth and during their children's early years. The results are reflected in lower levels of under-five mortality, reduced fertility, improved healthcare practices and later marriage and childbearing. Children – especially girls – born to educated mothers are more likely to attend school, resulting in a cycle of opportunity that extends across generations (UNICEF, 2016).

The key role of education in breaking the cycle of disadvantage is also emphasised in the 2013 EU Recommendation on Investing in Children, as high-quality education promotes children's emotional, social, cognitive and physical development (European Commission, 2013). The recommendation emphasises the need to target resources and opportunities towards the more disadvantaged, to recognise and address spatial disparities in the availability and quality of educational provision, to create an inclusive learning environment, to address barriers which stop or seriously hinder children from attending or completing school, to improve the performance of students with low basic skills, to develop and implement comprehensive policies to reduce early school leaving, to strengthen equality legislation. Because the Roma minority in Europe faces particularly high rates of poverty, the recommendation also insists on the need to prepare teachers for social diversity and to deploy special cultural mediators and role models to facilitate the integration of Roma and children with an immigrant background.

It is not just the quality and inclusiveness of schools that determine educational outcomes for children from disadvantaged backgrounds. Children's educational performance can be adversely affected by a number of the factors identified earlier, including growing up in overcrowded and substandard housing and unsafe environments, having inadequate nutrition, suffering from poor health and lack of access to health services, facing financial barriers to participation in education or (as explained further in the next section) having few informal learning opportunities due to lack of sport, recreational and cultural activities. Limited access to play, books and materials or, increasingly, to digital equipment and media can also be barriers. The level of education of parents, especially mothers, is a key factor in children's educational progress and thus support to parents to help them contribute best to their children's development is very important. Also, the extent of stability and security of the households where children are living is an important factor. In addition, the negative impact of domestic violence and its harmful impact on children's development has been strongly highlighted during the COVID-19 crisis. So, to ensure that children from disadvantaged backgrounds participate in and benefit as fully as possible from education it is essential to address the other barriers that can affect their participation. A comprehensive approach to combating child poverty is an essential part of tackling educational disadvantage and inequality.

Sport, culture and leisure activities

Impact of poverty on access to sport, culture and leisure activities

There is a strong correlation between growing up in poverty and limited access to sport, cultural and leisure activities. This matters because effective and affordable access to extra-curricular activities is just as essential as access to formal education to the ability for the child to flourish and reach his or her full potential. Although children from disadvantaged backgrounds may benefit more from participation in such activities than their more privileged peers (because the link between these activities and academic, psychological, social and behavioural outcomes is stronger for them), they tend in fact to participate less (European Commission, 2021b). Where there is inadequate provision of good-quality play, recreation, sporting and cultural facilities or where access is expensive, then children and their families from low-income backgrounds are likely to be excluded from opportunities to participate (Eurochild and EAPN, 2013).

On average for the EU as a whole, income-poor children are more than four times as likely to be deprived of leisure activities. The difference is negligible in all EU countries except in Finland (EU–SILC Users' Data Base, 2021, authors' calculations).

The lack of access to extra-curricular activities deprives children of safe facilities and informal learning opportunities. In the UK, the Child Poverty Action Group documented the significant difference that sport makes to young lives: it contributes to young people's health and, therefore, their development; it involves engaging with other young people in a positive way, thereby helping to avoid trouble; and it encourages concentration, motivation and other learning skills that help their education, as well as their working and social lives. However, they go on to highlight that young people living in disadvantaged areas face many barriers to participating in sport. These include 'poor health among low-income households [which] inhibits exercise, with parental ill health impacting directly on children's levels of physical activity'; limited free or affordable sporting opportunities outside school; lack of safe spaces in which to play; and 'poorer local environments [which] have fewer open spaces and lower controls over conditions' (Power, 2015).

Impact of access to sport, culture and leisure activities on children's future prospects and IGPP

Participation in sport, culture and leisure activities plays a key role in promoting the well-being and development of children, fostering resilience and broadening social networks and thus breaking the cycle of disadvantage. Some studies have shown, for example, that sport participation in childhood is positively correlated with adult labour market outcomes. This can possibly work through the development of both cognitive and non-cognitive skills via sport practice and the effect of sport not only on health and fitness but also on self-image, preferences over effort and the building of social networks (Cabane and Clark, 2015).

Employment opportunities

The link between poverty and poor access to decent employment is well established and is a major factor in perpetuating IGPP. Taking up decent employment that provides a living wage, allowing workers to support themselves and their families, is generally the best route out of poverty. Employment opportunities may be insufficient, however, even where the degrees and skills rise within the population (Narayan et al, 2018). Schooling that does not lead to better employment opportunities may be an important source of frustration, and discourage parents from investing in improving the education of their children, or young adults from acquiring qualifications. Moreover, even general improvements in the labour market may not benefit people facing socioeconomic disadvantage as much as other parts of the population: some estimates have found that at least 50% of the variability of lifetime earnings across individuals is due to attributes determined by age 18 (Heckman and Mosso, 2014, p 3), and most of these attributes are in fact already present at age 5 (Heckman, 2008, p 12).

Why is it that general economic progress leading to jobs creation will not necessarily translate into poverty reduction? Firstly, not all jobs are decent jobs. Because they often have lower educational levels and qualifications, people in poverty are more likely to stay poor even when in employment, whether formal or informal. Most of the people experiencing poverty in low-income countries are employed, but their labour does not allow them to rise above the poverty line (United Nations General Assembly, 2005, para 9). Globally, an estimated 327 million wage earners (including 152 million women) are paid at or below the applicable hourly minimum wage: this means one in five (19% of the total) wage earners are not paid even that minimum amount (ILO, 2020, pp 16–17).

Even when receiving minimum wages, low-income earners can end up in situations of precarity, owing to forced informal work and wage theft or arrears. People in poverty consulted by De Schutter in the African continent and in Latin America shared experiences of incomplete wage payments, unexpected fees and deceit by their employers. Low-income workers may also fear that joining a union will lead to job loss. This results in lower unionisation rates and, in turn, stagnating wages and worse working conditions. (De Schutter, 2021a)

Secondly, even in countries where the rate of informal employment is relatively low, it may be difficult for people in poverty to find a job. This is in part because of the importance of social connections for access to employment: friends, family or other acquaintances play a significant role in helping to identify and seize opportunities (Loury, 2006, p 299). In the US, seven in ten job openings are not published on public job sites; eight in ten are filled through professional networks and interpersonal connections (Kaufman, 2011; see also Granovetter, 1995). In France, 41% of job openings were filled in 2020 through the 'hidden job market' (Randstad, 2021).

Thirdly, the 'aspirations window' may play a role: for children facing socioeconomic disadvantage, a life free from the burden of poverty may be difficult to imagine (Appadurai, 2004). Half of children whose parents are in the managerial class become managers themselves, but only less than a quarter of children of manual workers have a chance to become managers. The reproduction of privilege in the world of work remains a reality. In the US and in Germany, almost half of the sons of rich fathers are in the top earnings quartile themselves (OECD, 2018a, pp 15, 186). In Canada, almost seven out of ten sons born to fathers belonging to the top 1% income earners had a job with an employer for which their father had also worked; in Denmark, a little over half of the sons of fathers at this level did so (Corak and Piraino, 2011).

The mechanisms already outlined in areas such as education and employment suggest that it is not income poverty alone, nor even the sources of disadvantage that are generally – though not necessarily – associated with low incomes (such as poor access to health, to nutrition, to housing or to education), that explain the perpetuation of poverty: inequality itself is a contributing factor. In other terms, the gap between low-income and higher-income households, or the unequal distribution of wealth within society, are specific obstacles to social mobility, additional to the difficult living conditions that low-income households experience.

Growing up in persistent poverty undermines self-confidence, reduces a sense that there are pathways out of poverty, leads to a lack of positive role models and thus undermines aspirations. This is especially true in more unequal societies. Initiatives, therefore, which help to build self-confidence and resilience, foster aspirations, provide positive role models and support and encourage children and young people to find pathways out of poverty can really help. In India, five types of social mobility-promoting organisations have been identified which help smart and hard-working children with backgrounds in poverty to aspire, and to achieve, superior career options and outcomes: they do this through coaching, mentorship, guidance, information provision and other means (Krishna and Agarwal, 2017). Examining rural Ethiopia, Bernard and colleagues highlight the positive potential of peer effects. They suggest that the viewing of documentaries of people of similar background as the viewers and who achieved agriculture and small-business success may foster and inspire important progress and change (Bernard et al, 2014). In Bombay, a long-term intervention by the non-governmental organisation Akanksha was successful in inculcating a sense of agency, control (self-efficacy) and aspirations (non-cognitive skills) among children and adolescents living in slums: Akanksha uses workshops, mentoring, drama, art and story-telling for these purposes. There is evidence of substantial impacts on both self-esteem and self-efficacy, as well as evidence of a smaller impact on life evaluation and aspirations. Furthermore, evidence shows that higher self-esteem and self-efficacy are linked with success in school-leaving examinations and initial labour market outcomes (Krishnan and Krutikova, 2013).

Yet, these efforts may face another obstacle: the discrimination that people in poverty face in everyday life, in their encounters with social services or officials, in their dealings with landlords or employers or in schools. Such discrimination is still poorly understood and insufficiently studied: it deserves to be much more central in the efforts to combat poverty.

Discrimination

Discrimination causes and perpetuates poverty: this is in part why poverty is concentrated among certain ethnic groups, affects women more than men, or people with disabilities more than people without disabilities. The most discussed and most extensively documented forms of discrimination are those that are based on certain characteristics such as ethnicity or migrant status. These reduce the life chances of children belonging to the groups concerned. Such classic forms of status-based discrimination also contribute to a large extent to creating horizontal inequalities and thus to the perpetuation of poverty among those groups. In addition however, *poverty itself* can be a source of discrimination, whether it has its source in negative stereotypes about people in poverty (an attitude sometimes referred to as 'povertyism'), or whether it is grounded in what Edmund Phelps and Kenneth Arrow popularised as 'statistical discrimination' (Phelps, 1972; Arrow, 1973; Aigner and Cain, 1977), in which discriminatory practices by decision makers mean that decisions can be made with less effort, based on generalisations about the relationship between poverty and ability. We refer to these two forms of discrimination, respectively, as 'status-based' and 'poverty-based': especially when combined, in what the literature describes as 'intersectional' discrimination, these forms of discrimination create significant barriers to equality of opportunities.

Status-based discrimination

Status-based discrimination has long been recognised as an important obstacle explaining the perpetuation of poverty. UNICEF and the Global Coalition to End Child Poverty, for instance, identify social stigma and discrimination as one of the most fundamental and often deeply rooted causes of child poverty. While different countries display differing forms of discrimination, examples of widely prevalent forms of discrimination that children experience are based on caste, ethnicity, gender and sexual orientation, HIV status, disability, refugee and migrant status, among many other context-specific factors (UNICEF and the Global Coalition to End Child Poverty, 2017).

In the EU, as reported by Eurochild and EAPN, children (and their parents) coming from an ethnic minority (especially Roma and Traveller children) or migrants are more likely to experience discrimination and racism and are at higher risk of experiencing poverty. They also may have difficulties obtaining equal access to services and facilities because their social and cultural needs are not sufficiently taken into account; or due to practical and administrative barriers or legal and structural discrimination on the basis of residence status (Eurochild and EAPN, 2013). The poor access of Roma and children with a migrant background to essential services is also highlighted in various EU countries (Frazer et al, 2020).

The link between poverty and race is also evident in the US. Wagmiller and Adelman report that:

> Nearly one-quarter of African-American children live in poverty for more than three-fourths of their childhood and more than one-third are poor for at least half of their childhood. On average, a white child spends only 8.9 percent of childhood living in poverty. By contrast, an African-American child is poor for nearly two-fifths of childhood on average. (Wagmiller and Adelman, 2009, p 3)

Noting that 'individuals who were poor during childhood are more likely to be poor as adults than are those who were never poor', they conclude that 'this is especially true for African-Americans', and also that 'racial disadvantages mean that mobility out of poverty for African-Americans is far more difficult than it is for whites' (Wagmiller and Adelman, 2009).

These children and their parents may also have more limited access to a broad range of social networks, which further reduces opportunities to move out of poverty and reduces social mobility. The loss of social contacts can be worst for those young people living in poverty who do not live with their families and are not able to do so, for example for unaccompanied-minor migrants or for some young people who have fled an unsafe family environment due to violence and/or abuse. Some may face a childhood of poverty, homelessness and insecurity (Eurochild and EAPN, 2013).

Poverty-based discrimination

Discrimination may thus cause poverty; but poverty itself can become the source of discrimination. When people in poverty are asked about their experience of poverty, they spontaneously refer to the humiliation and negative stereotyping they face in a number of settings: in their search for a job or for an apartment; in their interaction with schoolteachers or healthcare providers; or, of course, in their encounters with social workers and administrations.

The daily experience of discrimination and social and institutional maltreatment contributes to the vicious cycles in which they are trapped. Social discrimination was a major theme in the 'Voices of the Poor' study of 2000 (Narayan et al, 2000), and 'social maltreatment' is one of the 'hidden dimensions of poverty' highlighted in the study conducted jointly by Oxford University and by ATD Fourth World using the 'merging of knowledge' methodology ensuring involvement of people in poverty. In this latter study, 'social maltreatment' is described as 'the way in which people in poverty are typically treated within and by the community', often facing blame and stigma: 'The process of othering is commonplace in which people in poverty are thought to be different in kind and socially inferior, engaging in disreputable behaviour either as a cause or a result of their poverty.' Social maltreatment in turn feeds institutional maltreatment or abuse, defined as 'the common failure of public and private institutions to respond appropriately to the circumstances, needs and aspirations of people in poverty' (Bray et al, 2020).

Discrimination against people in poverty is thus a major obstacle to the eradication of poverty. It is an affront to human dignity as well as to the ideal of equal opportunities. It creates obstacles, additional to the lack of income, to access to employment, education, housing or social services. It may result in certain social goods or programmes not reaching people in poverty, due either to discriminatory treatment by public officials or private employers or landlords, or to the fear of maltreatment leading people in poverty themselves not to apply for a job, not to claim certain benefits or not to seek access to certain programmes. Discrimination may also lead people in poverty to lower their aspirations, whether for themselves or for their children, as to what they can achieve, thus leading to a reduced investment in education (Appadurai, 2004).

Normative instruments have gradually sought to respond. The 2005 Principles and Guidelines for a Human Rights Approach to Poverty Reduction Strategies describe poverty as a process in which the various deprivations are 'mutually reinforcing', and associated with 'stigma, discrimination, insecurity and social exclusion' (Office of the High Commissioner for Human Rights [OHCHR], Geneva, 2005, para 15). The 2012 Guiding Principles on Extreme Poverty and Human Rights, which the United Nations Human Rights Council adopted in September 2012, note that persons experiencing extreme poverty in particular 'live in a vicious cycle of powerlessness, stigmatisation, discrimination, exclusion and material deprivation, which all mutually reinforce one another'. In a fast-growing number of countries, the anti-discrimination framework includes a prohibition of discrimination on grounds of 'social origin', 'property', 'socio-economic condition' or simply 'poverty' or 'economic vulnerability'.

The fight against anti-poor prejudice is a long-term challenge, considering the widespread nature of povertyism. In France, a test relying on sending curriculum vitae (CVs) to employers showed a 30% net discrimination rate against candidates presenting a CV with indicators of poverty (such as an address in temporary housing shelter or previous employment in social enterprises) (ATD Fourth World, 2016). In Canada, a survey conducted by the Ontario Human Rights Commission showed that people experiencing poverty received more negative evaluations than any other group: only 39% of those surveyed had 'somewhat positive' feelings towards those receiving social assistance (McIsaac, 2018). Research conducted in the Netherlands showed how, in comparison to their higher-income peers, low-income students receive lower-quality advice from their teachers regarding the level of secondary education they should pursue, compared to the level of secondary education that is indicated by the standardised test at the end of primary school (Nederlands Jeugdinstituut, 2020).

Discrimination against people in poverty thus affects low-income individuals across all the areas that matter the most for social cohesion: it is, in that sense, systemic. Schools tend to reproduce inequalities and reward the codes acquired in better-off households: children from poor families face exclusion at school due to their social origin (OECD, 2019b, p 61), and participatory studies have illustrated that the shame experienced by children in poverty is one of the key obstacles to successful schooling (ATD Quart Monde and Changement pour l'Egalité, 2017), which compounds the disadvantage that children from lower socioeconomic status face because they are less well prepared for formal education: in France, for example, the difference in the PISA test outcomes between the richest and poorest students amounted to 115 points in the science performance, the equivalent of about three years of schooling (World Bank, 2018, p 78). As already noted, people living on low incomes also cluster in certain neighbourhoods where housing is affordable, but which are often less well connected to job opportunities and closer to sources of pollution (van Ham et al, 2014). The long-term unemployed and those who lack social connections experience the greatest difficulties in having access to employment, even when they have the right qualifications. Humiliating experiences with healthcare providers, combined with an inability to pay, may discourage people in poverty from seeking healthcare (Canvin et al, 2007).

The instances of discrimination in various spheres of life are mutually reinforcing. If they live in impoverished and remote neighbourhoods, people in poverty will face employers who will suspect that they are less reliable, since they have to travel longer distances to work; and their health may deteriorate as a result of a lack of access to green areas, which may reduce their productivity at work, thus further confirming the negative stereotypes of the employer. Children who face bullying at school because they don't have the right clothes, or who are ashamed of their parents, will drop out earlier from school, especially if they have no role models to relate to and if they anticipate that they will face discrimination in employment. These are self-reinforcing mechanisms that call for structural solutions.

Anti-poor prejudice is also systemic in that it is widespread, and may lead actors prone to discriminate to rationalise their behaviour as a response to attitudes of others. The employer may anticipate that clients expect to be served by an employee who has a good presentation and uses the right cultural codes. The school direction may be under the pressure of parents insisting that the school remains socially homogeneous. Residents of a particular neighbourhood may express the fear that the value of their property will fall if the neighbourhood becomes more diverse, which in turn puts pressure on landlords to rent only to tenants who will present the right 'fit' within the community. Moreover, discrimination within an organisation means that few people from a low-income background will be in decision-making positions: the decisions made may therefore be systematically skewed against people in poverty, whose specific life experiences will be ignored; and selection processes within the organisation may be based on co-optation and therefore reduce the opportunities of individuals with a different background.

It is perhaps in the sphere of employment that the ability of anti-poor prejudice to lead to self-reinforcing mechanisms entrenching discriminatory behaviour is both the most visible and the most pernicious. Facing prejudice leads people of lower socioeconomic status to invest less in the acquisition of qualifications that would allow them to have access to better-paid jobs: the more they are confronted with discrimination in the field of employment, the less they have an incentive to build human capital. Discrimination also results in a situation where people in poverty lack role models to which they can relate and that would allow them to build confidence (Lockwood and Kunda, 1997).

Indeed, even where people from a low-income background succeed in being employed, they will underperform if confronted with a manager who is biased against them, for example because the employer believes they are lazy (a common prejudice which long-term unemployed people encounter) (Van Belle et al, 2018), thus reinforcing further the negative prejudices of that manager: negative stereotypes against people from low-income backgrounds thus become self-fulfilling prophecies (Glover et al, 2017). This will be the case especially if they face what is called the 'stereotype threat' (that is, the fear of being judged and confirming negative stereotypes, undermining self-confidence [Cadinu et al, 2005]), which has been documented with respect both to ethnic minorities (Steele and Aronson, 1995) and to castes: in an experiment led in the Indian state of Uttar Pradesh, it was shown that the performance of 321 low-caste junior high school students on a maze-solving exercise (compared to that of 321 high-caste peers) was significantly lower when caste was publicly revealed, in other terms, when the results of the test could be interpreted as confirming caste stereotypes (Hoff and Pandey, 2006).

As a result of these entrenched mechanisms, negative stereotypes about people in poverty will not disappear on their own; nor will they be wiped out by markets alone. Indeed, what may initially be anti-poor prejudice based on false assumptions about the ability and reliability of people with low-income backgrounds may gradually turn into the kind of statistical discrimination already referred to (Phelps, 1972; Arrow, 1973; Aigner and Cain, 1977): anti-poor bias leads people from low-income backgrounds to underinvest in the acquisition of skills because they anticipate they will be harshly judged anyway, and this leads to negative stereotypes against them being reinforced, up to the point when they harden into statistical discrimination. In the case of long-term unemployed people, this is further reinforced by 'rational herding', that is, the assumption by prospective employers that a job-seeker must have been assessed by other employers and that there must be have been a reason why the candidate was not hired (Oberholzer-Gee, 2008).

Intra-household dynamics, gender and sacrifice

Gender and intra-household dynamics are also key factors influencing the perpetuation of poverty. Women tend to be disproportionately affected by poverty, and mothers also tend to play an influential role in determining whether this poverty is perpetuated into the next generation. In most contexts, girls' experience of poverty will differ from that of boys. Traditional child poverty measures, however, often do not effectively identify these differentiated experiences and impacts. Bringing in other analysis, listening to children, and specific indicators and indices (for example the Adolescent Girls Index in Uganda) can help to identify specific gendered vulnerabilities and policy responses (UNICEF and the Global Coalition to End Child Poverty, 2017).

Intra-household dynamics

The extent to which children are impacted upon by growing up in households living in poverty is significantly affected by intra-household dynamics and women's agency and empowerment. Women's own nutrition, health and well-being has a deep impact on child nutrition and well-being (Bird and Higgins, 2011). Strengthened economic bargaining power for women not only benefits their own well-being; it also increases spending on items which enhance the welfare of the household, such as education, food and health, while reducing expenditures on alcohol and cigarettes (Booysen and Guvuriro. 2021). While this is well documented in developing countries, it is also true in advanced economies. In the UK, for instance, the transfer of child allowances from husbands to wives in the decade 1970–80 had a positive impact on children's clothing and women's clothing (Lundberg et al, 1997).

Women's empowerment is also important for the child's well-being because of its impacts on the composition of the household. There is a correlation between the number of siblings and IGPP, because this affects the material and other resources available and distributed to individuals. Differences in resource allocation and access to nutrition and services within households can be explained by age, relationship to household head, gender or other forms of social difference such as sexuality or occupation (Bird and Higgins, 2011).

Gender

Children growing up in lone-parent households (the vast majority of which are headed by women) are particularly at risk of poverty. The risk is particularly important in rural areas and, of course, where the gender pay gap is important, or where women are disproportionately represented in atypical and uncertain forms of work contracts (zero-hours contracts, temporary work, interim jobs, part-time working), all factors that put women at greater risk of poverty. Based on these findings, a report of the European Parliament concludes that 'given the inter-generational dimensions of poverty, addressing the situation of girls and young women who are facing social exclusion and poverty is key to tackling the feminisation of poverty' (European Parliament, 2016).

Another key element that can contribute to IGPP is child marriage, which robs girls from their childhoods. UNICEF stresses that ending child marriage would mean that girls and women will have higher chances of making the most of their lives and giving their best to their households, communities and societies – 'which will go a long way towards breaking inter-generational cycles of poverty and strengthening communities and nations. Ending child marriage unlocks possibilities that can transform life for girls and yield benefits for us all' (UNICEF, 2016). Governments are just starting to wake up to this issue. In rural Bangladesh, an initiative to empower girls through conditional incentives for families of adolescent girls led to substantial reductions in child marriage and teenage childbearing in a setting with high rates of underage marriage; the impacts on educational attainment for girls in school were immediate and significant (Buchmann et al, 2018).

Sacrifice

Parents in poverty tend to sacrifice their own needs in order to avoid deprivation for their children (for example, Main and Bradshaw, 2016). At the same time, children living in poverty too often make sacrifices to support their households, such as dropping out of school early to begin to work or to care for household members. ATD Fourth World emphasises the extent to which such sacrifices damage their development and limit their opportunities to escape poverty. Children prioritise their household's needs – for instance, by agreeing to leave school or earning independently – while knowing the costs to their reputation and for their future. Missing school or falling behind in their studies is painful for children because they feel helpless in the face of low-quality teaching, parental workloads and discrimination. They also feel angry and frightened about their future because they see a good education as necessary to move out of poverty. Children also suffer on behalf of their parents, whom they love and they see are not coping. They experience related disempowerment (Main, 2018; Bray et al, 2019).

Environmental shocks, climate change and IGPP

Climate disruptions and related environmental shocks have a major impact on children's health, especially in developing countries. Environmental shocks can destroy water and sanitation infrastructure, exposing people to raw sewage; floods leaving behind stagnant water and the risk of cholera and malaria infection; food shortages, which are associated with lower levels of consumption and nutrition; and also violating the right to water and sanitation. People living in poverty are also more likely to lose their places of shelter and other assets as a result of environmental hazards, not least because they often have no choice but to live in areas that are regularly threatened by floods or mudslides (Akter and Mallick, 2013; Nguyen, 2016).

Climate change has negative effects on public infrastructure, socioeconomic and demographic inequality and physical and mental health outcomes. Children in poverty are at highest risk of experiencing these outcomes. Climate change increases the likelihood of wildfires, flooding and drought, which disproportionately harm poor children's material conditions by damaging the built environment and vital infrastructure. It exacerbates existing socioeconomic disparities in impoverished communities by impeding educational attainment, increasing poverty rates and reducing income stability. It impairs the physical and mental health of children, since in the aftermath of climate change-related events low-income children are more likely to suffer from malnutrition, vector-borne diseases, stress-induced mental illnesses and diseases stemming from air pollution and extreme heat.

This is how the Intergovernmental Panel on Climate Change (IPCC) describes the connections between climate change and poverty:

> Climatic variability and climate change are widely recognized as factors that may exacerbate poverty, particularly in countries and regions where poverty levels are high (Leichenko and Silva, 2014). The [Fifth Assessment Report (AR5)] noted that climate change-driven impacts often act as a threat multiplier in that the impacts of climate change compound other drivers of poverty (Olsson et al, 2014). Many vulnerable and poor people are dependent on activities such as agriculture that are highly susceptible to temperature increases and variability in precipitation patterns (Shiferaw et al, 2014; Miyan, 2015). Even modest changes in rainfall and temperature patterns can push marginalized people into poverty as they lack the means to recover from associated impacts. Extreme events, such as floods, droughts, and heat waves, especially when they occur in series, can significantly erode poor people's assets and further undermine their livelihoods in terms of labour productivity, housing, infrastructure and social networks (Olsson et al, 2014). (Allen et al, 2018, p 55)

A brief of the International Institute for Sustainable Development (IISD) on *Merging the Poverty and Environment Agendas* concludes: 'Eradicating poverty is directly linked to how we manage ecosystems and the goods and services they provide. Thus, policy makers must see environmental sustainability as a central objective to eradicating poverty' (Paul, 2021). At the same time, efforts of governments to mitigate climate change have not always sufficiently taken into account the impacts on people in poverty. As summarised by an OECD study: 'while mitigation measures designed to reduce greenhouse gas emissions can benefit poor children by improving health, boosting economic activity, and creating jobs, other measures can result in regressive distributional effects that disproportionately harm poor children and low-income communities' (Adrian et al, 2020). The objective of poverty eradication should therefore not only lead to putting climate change mitigation at the top of the political agenda; it should also guide these efforts to ensure that how climate change mitigation policies are designed contributes to reducing poverty and inequality.

Impact of IGPP on behaviour, aspirations, hope and agency

The factors already outlined may trap people in poverty, creating vicious cycles in which poverty becomes self-perpetuating. But that is not all. Immersion in an environment of poverty and social exclusion for a long time can also have a strong negative impact on people's aspirations, self-confidence and decision making. This may be a less visible but significant obstacle to escaping poverty. A 2021 report for the European Commission reviews the set of 'support measures' that can help to 'optimise existing capabilities and behaviours', allowing children and adults to overcome adverse circumstances. Among the crucial 'protective factors' that favour such resilience, the reports lists 'positive support from family and the school, and the presence of external support systems' (Cassio et al, 2021): it reviews approaches to education (including sport and the arts) that can be helpful; it examines how to support solid and secure attachment relationships; how to support the creation of aspirations; and how to help people set and achieve their goals in practice. Such measures seem to work best when they are integrated into a comprehensive framework, addressing together the needs of the parents and of their children.

PART II

Why should we care?

The perpetuation of poverty from one generation to the next matters not only to people in poverty; it should be a concern to us all. It has serious economic, social and environmental consequences that are bad for everyone. We examine these consequences in more detail in Chapter Three.

THREE

Why IGPP is bad for all

Ending IGPP will greatly increase our ability to build a more inclusive, sustainable and peaceful world. It is no coincidence that ending poverty is goal 1 of the UN's Sustainable Development Goals (SDGs), agreed in 2015. This is not only because of the damage IGPP does to children, and it is not only because IGPP can be seen as a violation of human rights. It is also because of the damage it does to society and the dangers it creates for all our futures – endangering educational achievement, general health, skills, labour productivity and economic growth, social cohesion and social capital (that is, the trust that exists between the members of the community and thus their ability to work together to achieve social transformation), as well as the environment (UNICEF and the Global Coalition to End Child Poverty, 2017). In other words, there are serious social, economic and environmental costs to society that result from a failure to address IGPP, and these consequences greatly reduce our ability to address the major challenges we face if we are to build a better future for us all.

IGPP:

- undermines social solidarity and cohesion;
- has high economic costs and reduces economic productivity;
- increases social costs;
- increases family insecurity; and
- damages the environment and undermines efforts to create a sustainable future.

Social solidarity and cohesion undermined

Continuing poverty and persistent inequality undermine the social fabric. People are trapped in their low-income status and feel unable to improve their lives. In contrast, when people know that they have the opportunity to improve the lot of their family as compared to previous generations, this has a positive influence on life satisfaction and well-being, and it enhances a sense of social solidarity. Indeed, even high levels of inequality can seem tolerable to people if they perceive such a situation as transitory – if, to borrow from the metaphor put forward initially by Albert Hirschman and Michael Rothschild, the driver stuck in traffic sees the lane next to his own moving forward, he sees this with relief as an indication that he too, in time, shall benefit from the general progress (Hirschman and Rothschild, 1973). In contrast, where the individual perceives himself to be trapped in poverty, with few prospects for escaping from it, high inequality may lead to resentment: what was an uncomfortable but temporary gap becomes an insurmountable chasm, and the source of despair. In fact, this is precisely the sort of despair that Ann Case and Angus Deaton document among White Americans without a college degree whose life expectancy has been diminishing in the 21st century as a result of high suicide rates and drug and alcohol abuse: it is the despair of those who have lost hope in their ability to shape a better future for themselves and their children (Case and Deaton, 2020).

The psychological impacts of poverty traps are therefore real; they may be said to be deadly. Beyond the impacts on the well-being of the individual, however, poverty and inequality have impacts on society as a whole.

First, inequality leads to a form of 'modernisation of poverty' by creating new desires, leaving those whose purchasing power is comparatively lower than that of the rest of society in a state of permanent dissatisfaction. This is because inequality stimulates status competition and, thus, forms of material consumption by which individuals seek to signal their affiliation to particular social classes. We 'want' material things, for the most part, not merely because of the comfort they provide, but for the message we send to those around us by owning or using them. This was a key insight of Veblen in his *Theory of the Leisure Class*: 'the standard of expenditure which commonly guides our efforts', he wrote more than a century ago,

> is not the average, ordinary expenditure already achieved; it is an ideal of consumption that lies just beyond our reach, or to reach which requires some strain. The motive is emulation – the stimulus of an invidious comparison which prompts us to outdo those with whom we are in the habit of classing ourselves. (Veblen, 1899, p 64)

Since 'each class envies and emulates the class next above it in the social scale, while it rarely compares itself with those below or with those who are considerably in advance' (Veblen, 1899, p 64), unequal societies lead to a permanent race for status through consumption: social psychology has demonstrated that we attach more importance to our position in comparison to others against whom we rank ourselves, than to our absolute levels of consumption alone (Solnick and Hemenway, 1998; Dolan et al, 2008). The result is that, as noted by Tim Jackson, unless it is combined with greater equality, income growth is a 'zero-sum game': a growth in average incomes that would leave people as wide apart from one another would hardly satisfy their desire to compare favourably to those around them, and the gains in life satisfaction would be, at best, minimal (Jackson, 2017, p 57; Wilkinson and Pickett, 2018, p 226).

This may be called the counter-productivity of growth: at the same time that growth can allow economic progress, it also results in the emergence of new desires, quickly mistaken as needs, but the lack of fulfilment of which gives rise to new forms of exclusion. The more societies grow affluent, the more such social exclusion has its source in such a modernisation of poverty: even when the basic needs of an individual are satisfied, they remain socially excluded because social expectations rise with the increase in general affluence. In all but the poorest countries today, you are considered to be poor when you cannot afford a mobile phone, when you have no access to the internet, when you cannot organise a decent funeral for your parents or a decent wedding for your children or when you cannot face expenditures following catastrophic events such as the loss of a job or an illness. Poverty is not just the result of being unable to satisfy basic needs; it is the result of being unable to meet the expectations of neighbours or family. It is not an absolute notion; it is relative to the standard of living of others. It cannot be addressed solely by providing individuals with a minimum set of guarantees, by placing a roof over their heads or by putting food on their plates: it can be tackled only by combating the gaps between the richest and the poorest, and thus the social exclusion that results from social comparisons.

Tackling income and wealth inequalities is also important in order to avoid political disempowerment of people in poverty, and thus, in turn, a lack of responsiveness by the political decision-making system to the circumstances they face. The higher the level of inequality, the more participation in civic and political life by ordinary people, particularly among low-income groups, is discouraged (Alesina and La Ferrara, 2000; Uslaner and Brown, 2005). Members of such groups have fewer resources to spend on participation in civic life: they lack time, they face high opportunity costs and they have a low level of trust in their ability to make a difference. The result is a form of retreat from civic and political life, which soon creates a vicious cycle: as the cultural elites and high-income groups dominate the political scene, members of low-income groups are further unwilling to invest in a sphere which they feel is unresponsive to their needs and aspirations. In addition, the higher the level of inequality within society, the less its members see themselves as sharing common goals with others, which constitutes a further disincentive to civic participation (Rothstein and Uslaner, 2005).

There is ample research demonstrating that, even in the best-functioning democracies, the wealthiest groups of the population exercise a disproportionate influence in the political system (Gilens, 2012), and that this phenomenon has become worse with the growth of inequalities since the early 1980s: a study covering 136 countries for the period 1981–2011 showed that 'as income inequality increases, rich people enjoy greater political power and respect for civil liberties than poor people do' (Cole, 2018). It appears, thus, that civic and political participation will be lower among low-income groups, due to a lack of resources, and that it will be lower in more unequal societies, due to the fact that the 'common good' is less clearly identifiable in more stratified societies.

Researchers have sought to quantify the respective importance of both phenomena. In 2006, based on a survey of 137,000 individuals in 24 European countries, Bram Lancee and Herman van de Werfhorst sought to measure the relationship between levels of inequality and civic participation for different income groups, taking into account also the fact that the resources available for participation may result from various forms of support provided by the welfare state – such as subsidies for associations (Lancee and van de Werfhorst, 2011). Civic participation was measured on the basis of five criteria: participation in civic or neighbourhood associations, environmental groups and so forth; dedication of voluntary time to charitable causes; participation in recreational groups or associations such as sports clubs and so forth; involvement in political parties or associations or in trade unions; finally, participation in professional organisations.

The survey confirmed a close inverse correlation between the level of inequality and the degree of civic participation even apart from the resources available to individuals. Lancee and van de Werfhorst conclude that

> besides individual resources (income, education), more inequality at the top is associated with a lower likelihood to be active in a voluntary organization. ... [T]he depressing effect of above-median inequality on participation is invariant across income groups. Or, in other words, the association between income and civic participation is not dependent on the level of above-median income inequality. (Lancee and van de Werfhorst, 2011, p 29)

Nor is it significantly influenced by the provision of social services that increase the availability of resources, in particular for low-income groups. At the same time, 'the positive effect of below-median equality on civic participation is stronger for low-income households than for high-income households' (Lancee and van de Werfhorst, 2011, p 29): in other terms, it is primarily low-income groups whose degree of civic participation, including participation in political life, will increase following a reduction in inequality levels.

High economic costs, reduced economic productivity and increased social costs

The damaging economic and social impacts of poverty on society are particularly evident in the case of children. According to some estimates, poverty and associated health, nutrition and social factors prevent at least 200 million children in developing countries from attaining their development potential (UNICEF and the Global Coalition to End Child Poverty, 2017). This has long-term implications for economies and societies. Economic productivity is reduced as a result of economic inefficiency and waste of human resources/potential. Child poverty results in unrealised human potential and the misallocation of resources, as people's talents are wasted, or not developed, and disadvantaged households are excluded from opportunities that favour those born in greater privilege. In the US, McLaughlin and Rank have estimated that the economic cost of child poverty was 5.4% of GDP in 2015 (McLaughlin and Rank, 2018). These costs are linked to the loss of economic productivity, increased health and crime costs and increased costs because of child homelessness and maltreatment. In addition, they estimate that for every dollar spent on reducing childhood poverty, the country would save at least seven dollars spent on addressing the economic costs of poverty. UNICEF and the Global Coalition to End Child Poverty point out that while there is no research on this area in all regions, an estimate of the economic costs of child poverty in the US finds that the lost productivity and extra health and crime costs stemming from child poverty add up to roughly US$500 billion a year, or 3.8% of GDP (UNICEF and the Global Coalition to End Child Poverty, 2017). In the UK, the Joseph Rowntree Foundation has estimated that through a combination of public spending to deal with the fallout of child poverty on personal social services, school education and police and criminal justice and the annual cost of below-average employment rates and earnings levels among adults who grew up in poverty, child poverty costs the country at least £25 billion a year, including £17 billion that could accrue to the exchequer if child poverty were eradicated; this is equivalent to about 2% of GDP (Hirsch, 2008).

The impact of poverty on education inequalities is one factor in reduced economic productivity. One study by Hanushek and Woessmann seeks to quantify for the EU countries the economic benefits of educational improvement for low-performing students (as measured by the OECD's PISA survey[1]). They conclude that bringing all low-performing students up to the basic skill requirements (level 2 on the PISA tests) would boost average EU GDP over the 21st century by nearly 4% (with larger improvements in Member States with more low-skilled students) (Hanushek and Woessmann, 2019).

Child poverty results in poor health, higher levels of unemployment, more precarious employment and so forth – all of which lead to increased demands on public services (especially health and social welfare and social protection services), which provide a costly way to treat the symptoms as if to compensate our inability to treat the causes. More positively, the evidence in the US shows that the return on spending on children is high and that direct investment in low-income children's health and education is particularly effective (Hendren and Sprung-Keyser, 2020). Similarly, cost-benefit analyses show that providing secure housing to homeless people is generally cheaper than doing nothing, as homelessness has a large public cost in terms of health assistance, emergency support and complex interventions (Guio et al, 2021).

Rise in family insecurity

Bringing up children in poverty increases stress on families. Parents living in poverty face a daily struggle for survival for their families and are forced to make sacrifices to protect their children from the worst effects of poverty (Eurochild and EAPN, 2013). The stresses associated with poverty can be a key factor in increased family insecurity and break-up, and in the risk of children being brought up in institutions or of families feeling forced to entrust their children to others. The UN Committee on the Rights of the Child regularly insists that children have the right to grow up in families, and there is

---

[1] www.oecd.org/pisa/

clear evidence of the damage done by bringing up children in institutional settings and not in strong family and community settings (Lerch and Nordenmark Severinsson, 2019). This means that a key element in supporting children in poverty is supporting the security and well-being of their families, as has been well emphasised in Europe by the Confederation of Family Organisations in the EU (COFACE, 2020a) and globally by ATD Fourth World (ATD Fourth World, 2004).

Efforts to achieve an environmentally sustainable future undermined

As we outlined in Chapter Two, climate change and environmental shocks are an important factor in causing and perpetuating poverty, but the reverse is also true: poverty and inequality contribute to climate change and limit our ability to combat it. This complex relationship between poverty and the environment is well summed up by Niranjan Dev Bharadwaj in a blog for Voices of Youth (UNICEF's community for youth, by youth). He writes that:

Poverty often causes people to put relatively more pressure on the environment which results in larger families (due to high death rates and insecurity), improper human waste disposal leading to unhealthy living conditions, more pressure on fragile land to meet their needs, overexploitation of natural resources and more deforestation. Insufficient knowledge about agricultural practices can also lead to a decline in crop yield and productivity etc. ... [At the same time,] environmental problems add more to the miseries of poor people. Environmental problems cause more suffering among them as environmental damage increases the impact of floods and other environmental catastrophes. Soil erosion, land degradation and deforestation lead[ing] to a decline in food production along with a shortage of wood for fuel contribute to inflation. In short, the

> worst consequences of environmental deterioration,
> whether they be economical, social, or related to mental
> or physical wellbeing, are experienced by poor people.
> (Bharadwaj, 2016)

Thus, not only is the situation of people in poverty worsened by climate change but ongoing poverty is also an important factor increasing climate change and limiting our ability to tackle it and to create an environmentally sustainable future for us all.

The emerging ecosocial approach argues that inequality and environment degradation are different sides of the same coin and that we need to progress equality and environmental sustainability as interlinked goals. Achievement of each form of sustainability depends on the other and this understanding informs ecosocial ambition, analysis, solutions, and strategies for action (Murphy, 2023). We would agree that the persistence of inequality is itself a major obstacle to the ecological transformation. Indeed, we would argue that in order to accelerate the shift towards low-carbon societies and to combat the erosion of biodiversity, the fight against inequalities, rather than the pursuit of economic growth followed by redistribution of its outcomes, should take priority. The link is obvious at the macro level, once we consider that the more the wealth created is spread equally across the population, the easier it will be to reconcile the minimisation of environmental impacts with poverty-reduction objectives: if the benefits of increased prosperity trickle down to the worse-off in society, less growth will be required for the basic needs of all to be met. And since growing the economy cannot be done without increasing the use of resources and the production of waste, including greenhouse gas emissions responsible for climate disruptions, it is imperative that, where the economy still must grow (where poverty reduction depends on the further creation of wealth), it does so in ways that will maximise its positive impacts on lifting people out of poverty and that will minimise its ecological impacts.

Beyond that macro-level relationship between 'inclusive' growth and the ecological transformation, our conviction that the reduction of inequalities should be at the heart of the ecological transformation is based on two additional arguments. First, in more unequal societies, status anxiety is high, because rank, by definition, matters more in such societies in which differences between individuals or households are more pronounced. Unequal societies therefore cause a specific type of stress: individuals fear that they will fall from one rank to the next, as a result of which they adopt a competitive attitude which consists in the quest for status above other objectives, at the expense both of their individual health and of social capital. A 2007 cross-national survey of over 34,000 individuals carried out in 31 European countries thus showed that respondents from low-inequality countries reported less status anxiety (in response to the statement 'some people look down on me because of my job situation or income') than those in higher-inequality countries at all points on the income-rank curve (Layte and Whelan, 2014). Indeed, in unequal societies, 'status-seeking' (which includes concerns about relative social position, awareness of social hierarchies and an assessment of how much the person relies on the opinions of other people) (Paskov et al, 2017) is more frequent and widespread that in more equal societies: where there is inequality, there is constant social comparison, and there is a reduced sense of commonality and solidarity. This in turn encourages the kind of 'conspicuous consumption' referred to earlier, which is driven by a concern for social status, rather than by the requirement to satisfy the individual's basic needs.

Second, the use of resources is more efficient in more equal societies. Markets don't respond to needs. What they register is *demand*, as expressed in the purchasing power of consumers, in proportion to their ability to pay. Scitovsky therefore compared the marketplace to a plutocracy: it is 'the rule of the rich', he wrote, 'where each consumer's influence on what gets produced depends on how much he spends' (Scitovsky,

1992 [1976], p 8). Yet, once you get to vote on the allocation of resources in proportion to the money you can put on the table, it is our sense of priorities that gets distorted. In unequal societies, the 'desires' of the most affluent may take precedence over the satisfaction of basic needs linked to housing, health, education or access to green areas for the least affluent. Greater equality mitigates this distortion.

Designing pro-poor policies and combating inequality can therefore serve to mitigate the tension between ecological sustainability and poverty reduction, and ensure that whatever economic growth there is shall effectively improve the situation of people in poverty, rather than fuel consumption by the rich.

PART III

What can be done?

The vicious cycles that perpetuate poverty can be broken. The question is neither one of sufficient resources nor one of lack of solutions: what is needed is a combination of political imagination and political will. The following two chapters explore the range of policies that should be put in place to accelerate the fight against poverty. Chapter Four explores the potential of classic tax-and-transfer policies on which the welfare state was built. Since the early 20th century, poverty was addressed through a combination of progressive taxation and redistributive welfare schemes, including investments in ECEC and other essential services. This effort must continue. Indeed, more than ever, with the rise of the levels of public debt, we are facing the threat of welfare state retrenchment: to combat poverty, a first priority should be to avoid the dismantling of what we already have, and move towards the universalisation of social protection floors.

The old recipes will not be sufficient, however. We should also explore how to combat poverty without growth, by making the market more inclusive: avoiding exclusion in the first place, rather than compensating post hoc for the exclusionary impacts of markets as they have developed. This means guaranteeing the right to work, against the fate of structural unemployment. It means providing all young adults, unconditionally, with a basic income, to move closer towards the ideal of a society in which all individuals start with equal opportunities, independent, in particular, from the wealth of their parents. And it means prohibiting discrimination on grounds of socioeconomic disadvantage. Chapter Five explores these tools. What they have in common is that they seek to shape an inclusive economy: one that prevents social exclusion, rather than seeking to boost growth to remedy the exclusionary impacts of an insufficiently shared development process.

FOUR

Post-market redistribution

The classic approach to combating poverty has relied on economic growth, combined with tax-and-transfer schemes. Although pursuing economic growth at all costs is neither realistic nor sustainable, due to the impacts of growth on resource use and the waste and pollution it leads to, the social protection provided by the welfare state still provides an important bulwark against poverty and social exclusion. And while this approach to poverty reduction will not suffice, it remains essential, in combination with other measures (including the gradual transformation of the welfare State in order to reduce its dependence on growth), in the short term. We identify four priorities in this regard.

Mobilising resources to combat poverty: the role of taxation schemes

Widening the tax base to ensure adequate funding for the fight against poverty

In order to finance social protection, it is first necessary that countries increase the mobilisation of domestic resources, by expanding the tax base on which they rely. For many years, the dominant view was that low-income countries were unable to achieve this. In 2009, basing himself on data from 2000–05, Martin Ravallion famously arrived at the conclusion that only by imposing 'prohibitive' tax rates (of 60% and above, and often beyond 100%) on the relatively rich (that is, on those whose incomes exceed US$13 per day in 2005 PPP, which corresponds to the level of consumption defining the poverty line in rich countries) would it be possible for low-income countries to effectively end poverty. In other terms: although various other measures might be relied on to reduce poverty in these countries, poverty was considered to be so widespread, and wealth creation so woefully insufficient, that taxation was not a promising way to achieve this objective (Ravallion, 2009). The implication was that, for these poor countries, redistribution of wealth was not a substitute for economic growth and international support: before wealth could be redistributed, there needed to be wealth to share.

Some 20 years have passed, however, during which economic growth has been strong for most of the countries of this group: subsequent research, using a methodology very similar to that of Ravallion, has come to the conclusion that 'most developing countries [now] have the financial scope to dramatically speed up the end of poverty based on national capacities at the global poverty lines of $1.90 or the $2.50 line' (Hoy and Sumner, 2016, p 19). That means an untapped potential. In many countries, particularly developing countries, the tax base is very low, and does not allow the states concerned to mobilise sufficient resources for the deployment of social protection. Inter-regional differences are huge in this area: it was estimated in 2013, for instance, that in developed countries, revenue from personal income tax is 8.4% of GDP, whereas in Latin American countries, for instance, this tax generates only 1.4% of GDP (Corbacho et al, 2013, p 115).[1] It has been

---

[1] This discrepancy, as a measure of the degree of progressivity of the tax system (that is, of its ability to reduce inequalities) is hardly attenuated by taking into account the proportion of the personal income tax represented in the total tax burden: by 2013, the total tax burden represented 34.8% of the GDP in OECD countries, and it was 23.4% in Latin America

noted that 'if all developing countries were able to raise 15% of their national income in tax, a commonly accepted minimum figure (the OECD average is 37%), they could realise at least an additional $198 billion per year, more than all foreign development assistance combined' (Sepulveda, 2014, para 56).

A specific area in which action could be taken to widen the tax base in order to fund the realisation of social rights is by reducing, or eliminating entirely, favourable fiscal treatment granted to foreign investors in order to attract capital. There is in fact ample evidence that such 'tax holidays' or even, more generally, legal protections granted to investors, have little or no impact on the ability of the country to attract investment (De Schutter et al, 2012). The major determinants of foreign direct investment are economic factors such as market size and trade openness, as measured by exports and imports in relation to total GDP. For other variables there is less consensus in the literature. In general, the studies find that the political and economic factors such as market size, skilled labour and trade policies are more important for the locational decision of foreign investment than the legal structure for protection of investors' rights and the ability to avoid double taxation by double-taxation treaties: there is weak evidence that the conclusion of investment agreements guaranteeing extensive rights to investors has more than a marginal impact on foreign direct investment inflows, and where it does seem to have some effect, it is mostly as a substitute for poor institutional quality, particularly in sub-Saharan African countries or in transition economies swiftly moving towards open market policies (Sornarajah, 1986; Jackee, 2011).

Studies on the locational choices of investors tend to show that the levels of taxes paid by corporations play only a minor role in the decisions of investors concerning the location of

---

(Corbacha et al, 2013). Therefore, the personal income tax represented about one quarter of the tax burden in OECD countries, but only 5.98% of the tax burden in Latin American countries.

their investment. Yet, the myth persists that attracting investors by lowering the corporate tax base is a sustainable strategy, as if the comparative advantage of countries could be maintained by them continuing to be unable to educate a highly-qualified workforce, to maintain well-functioning public services and to improve the quality of life for those working under their jurisdiction. Fiscal competition persists between jurisdictions. The result is that we have fiscal policies that, instead of shifting more of the tax burden onto the wealthiest corporations and the richest individuals, as both economic common sense and human rights would require, end up taxing wage earners and consumers through value added tax (VAT) and the imposition of users' fees in sectors such as health or education. According to calculations of the World Bank, the average total tax rate payable by businesses on their commercial profits decreased from 53.5% to 40.8% between 2005 and 2015, and has stabilised since.[2] Although some countries moved in the opposite direction (Argentina and Chile are examples in Latin America; Malaysia and Niger provide illustrations in Asia and in Africa), the trend downwards is massive: for many countries, the reduction of corporate taxes is measured in double digits. On average, the total tax rates in the euro area countries went from 51.0% to 43.6%, a trend corresponding roughly to the tendency in the EU as a whole. But the phenomenon is

---

[2] This is a non-weighted average: small economies count as much as large ones in the calculation of the average. The total tax rate, for the purpose of this calculation, is the 'amount of taxes and mandatory contributions payable by businesses after accounting for allowable deductions and exemptions as a share of commercial profits'. For more details, see http://data.worldbank.org/indicator/IC.TAX.TOTL.CP.ZS?end=2015&start=2005&view=chart (last consulted on 22 November 2022). Some countries have lowered corporate taxes faster than others: during this ten-year period of fiscal competition (2005–15), Albania lowered corporate taxes from 58.2% to 36.5%, Belarus from 137.3% to 51.8% and Uzbekistan from 96.7% to 41.1%; Canada went from 47.5% to 21.1%, and Paraguay from 54.5% to 35.0%. Turkey moved from 52.8% to 40.9%.

especially spectacular in the countries classified by the UN as least developed, where the rate went down on average from 75.4% to 44.7%; if we consider heavily indebted poor countries alone, the decrease is from 81.2% to 52.7%.

Whether they focus on corporate income tax rates or on the protection of investors' rights through investment treaties or double-taxation treaties, the lesson from these studies on investors' locational choices is clear: if there is one means through which revenues from taxation could increase rather painlessly (and at a relatively low administrative cost), it is by raising the taxes owed by foreign corporations operating in the country, or by closing loopholes, such as price transfer mechanisms, allowing such corporations to escape local taxes if not entirely, at least to a very large extent. The global minimum effective corporate tax rate of 15%, as proposed under Pillar II of the OECD Two Pillar Solution, is a step in this direction: although various studies show that the benefits, particularly for African countries, are likely to be minimal (see, for example, Coulibaly, 2022), this global effort at least should slow down the 'race to the bottom' in corporate taxation, which ultimately is damaging to the ability of all countries to finance their development.

Implementing progressive tax policies

The second requirement for a financing of social protection is to move to a more progressive taxation system. A former UN Special Rapporteur on extreme poverty and human rights argued that states should be encouraged to

> set up a progressive tax system with real redistributive capacity that preserves, and progressively increases, the income of poorer households. ... [A]ffirmative action measures aimed at assisting the most disadvantaged individuals and groups that have suffered from historical or persistent discrimination, such as well-designed subsidies or tax exemptions, would not be discriminatory. In contrast,

a flat tax whereby all people are required to pay an equal proportion of their income would not be conducive in achieving substantive equality, as it limits the redistributive function of taxation. (Sepulveda, 2014, para 16)

Her successor in the mandate, Philip Alston, emphasised this point further, regretting that we are still far from 'recognising the fact that tax policy is, in many respects, human rights policy', despite the obvious contribution taxation makes to the fulfilment of human rights: 'The regressive or progressive nature of a State's tax structure, and the groups and purposes for which it gives exemptions or deductions, shapes the allocation of income and assets across the population, and thereby affects levels of inequality and human rights enjoyment' (Alston, 2015, para 53). It is time that these calls be heeded.

The need for more progressive tax policies is further highlighted by the extent to which the wealthiest have captured a disproportionate part of economic growth. Christensen et al (2023) have calculated that the richest 1% grabbed nearly two-thirds of all new wealth, worth US$42 trillion, created since 2020, almost twice as much money as the bottom 99% of the world's population. They present an analysis by the Fight Inequality Alliance, Institute for Policy Studies, Oxfam and the Patriotic Millionaires, of the impact of an annual wealth tax of up to 5% on the world's multi-millionaires and billionaires. Such a tax could raise US$1.7 trillion a year – enough to lift two billion people out of poverty, fully fund the shortfalls on existing humanitarian appeals, deliver a ten-year plan to end hunger, support poorer countries being ravaged by climate impacts and deliver universal healthcare and social protection for everyone living in low- and lower-middle-income countries.

Progressivity of taxation as a human rights requirement

Redistributive fiscal policies and social spending, particularly on social security, have had a major role to play to reduce the

Figure 4.1: Impacts on inequality (measured as Gini coefficient) of tax-benefit systems relative to market plus pension income, overall population, in 2017, for 16 European OECD countries

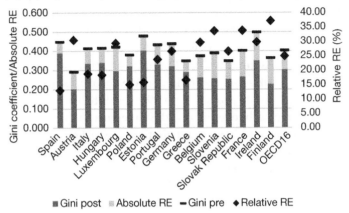

■ Gini post　▨ Absolute RE　━ Gini pre　◆ Relative RE

Note: 'Gini pre' refers to the Gini coefficients resulting from incomes from market and pensions before redistribution. 'Gini post' refers to the Gini coefficients after redistribution following taxes and transfers. The absolute redistributive effects ('Absolute RE', left vertical axis) of tax-benefit systems are calculated as the difference between a 'pre-Gini' (that is, inequality before taxes and transfers) and a 'post-Gini' (that is, inequality after taxes and transfers). The 'Relative RE' (right vertical axis) refers to the redistributive effects as a percentage of the 'pre-Gini' incomes. 'OECD16' refers to the average across the 16 European OECD countries. Source: OECD, 2021b, p 32, Figure 7, Panel A.

levels of inequality that would result from market incomes for different groups of the population. In OECD countries, public cash transfers, together with income taxes and social security contributions, were estimated to reduce inequality among the working-age population (measured by the Gini coefficient) by an average of about one quarter across OECD countries during the period from the mid-1980s to the late 2000s (OECD, 2011). Figure 4.1 illustrates the contribution of redistributive public policies to the reduction of inequalities.

Comparing inequality levels based on market incomes (combined with pension) with inequality levels following redistribution through taxes and social security, the figure shows that, while Gini coefficients before redistribution range between 0.498 in Ireland and 0.292 in Austria, after redistribution they lie between 0.403 in Estonia and 0.203 in Austria. As in the OECD study of 2011 referred to earlier, redistribution results in a decrease of inequality by, on average, about a quarter (0.099 absolute Gini points). Absolute redistributive effects (the difference between 'pre-redistribution' and 'post-redistribution' inequality levels) are high for Ireland (0.148) and low for Poland (0.057), Greece (0.058) and Spain (0.058). In relative terms, that is, relative to the absolute level of incomes, Finnish taxes and benefits are the most redistributive ones (37.2%) and Spanish ones the least (13%) (OECD, 2021b).

A progressive tax system can help to combat poverty in two ways: first, by reducing post-tax levels of income inequality; and second, by increasing the fiscal capacity of the state, thereby allowing it to provide the population with services in areas such as education, health, housing or public transportation. It can therefore contribute to reducing the impact on low-income households of income and wealth disparities. Three remarks are in order, however.

First, it is important to relate progressivity in taxation schemes to the scope and content of the redistributive policies adopted within each country. A progressive tax system can have an impact on the reduction of inequalities only if the revenue from the taxes collected is redistributed through social policies that benefit the poor, rather than being spent on investments that will only allow the rich to become richer. For the effective realisation of economic, social and cultural rights, it is the *combination* of revenue mobilisation and of spending choices that matters, and neither of these two elements alone will in itself suffice to assess whether the efforts of the state are sufficient: just as one can easily imagine a state with generous social policies addressed at tackling poverty, but in which such policies are essentially financed by the poor themselves (see, for instance, De Schutter, 2010, para 36), it is also possible to have a state that taxes the rich but does not use the revenues collected in ways that have a significant impact on the reduction of inequalities.

Second, the ability for even a progressive tax system to reduce inequalities depends not only on the contribution of the richest part of the population to public revenue in *percentage* terms, but also on the *absolute* levels of such contributions: if, for example, the richest decile of the population pays 90% of the total income taxes collected in the country, the taxation system may be said to be progressive according to the most common measure of tax progressivity, known as the Kakwani index (Kakwani, 1977). But if those richest 10% are taxed at very low rates, the redistributive capacity of the taxation remains very limited: such a redistributive capacity is captured by another index, known as the Reynolds–Smolensky index, which measures the difference in income distribution before and after the tax is imposed (Reynolds and Smolensky, 1977; Haughton and Khandker, 2009). The Kakwani index basically measures how much the rich contribute to state revenue; the Reynolds–Smolensky index measures how much the poor benefit. One important consequence of the distinction between these measures is that a tax reform that may at first appear as regressive because the *proportion of the total tax revenue paid by the richest part of the population* will decrease (leading, in other terms, the effort to be spread across a larger part of the population), nevertheless may have progressive consequences if the *overall tax rates* and thus the revenue the state may mobilise are increased.

Third, the introduction of a progressive taxation scheme could have counter-productive impacts if it resulted in choking the economy and significantly slowing down economic activity, thus, in the medium to long term, destroying the very revenue base the state may be able to count on in order to finance its social policies. Indeed, a limitation common to the Kakwani and Reynolds-Smolensky indexes is that neither of them takes into account, in a dynamic perspective, the changes in revenue that may result from the introduction of tax reforms (Díaz de Sarralde et al, 2010). This, however, is an area in which the persistence of certain myths often has made a disservice to public debate. One assumption in particular, popularised as the 'Kuznets curve', is that the growth of inequality is an inevitable price to pay for economic growth, so that the introduction of policies to combat inequalities, if it occurs too early, might damage the prospects for development. However, quite apart from the fact that the original reasoning of Simon Kuznets, which applied to fast-growing nations going through rapid processes of industrialisation and urbanisation (Kuznets, 1955), could not be transposed to advanced industrial economies in which these processes are completed, the ideological uses made of his work do not correspond to the actual findings of Kuznets: whereas there may have been, historically, a correlation between the structural transformation linked to industrialisation and the increase of inequality, it does not follow that such increase should be treated as a condition for industrialisation – indeed, one may suspect that industrialisation would have been far less damaging to social cohesion, and thus far more sustainable, with robust redistributive schemes compensating the losers by transferring resources from the gainers. Nor, indeed, do such ideological uses have any (other) solid data to rely on. Quite to the contrary in fact, there is now a consensus that high levels of taxation, allowing the state to adopt robust redistributive policies and provide high-quality public services, far from being an obstacle to economic growth, are an indispensable ingredient thereof: the International Monetary Fund (IMF) found that 'the combined direct and indirect effects of redistribution, including the growth effects of the resulting lower inequality, are on average pro-growth' (Ostry et al, 2014; also Berg and Ostry, 2011). Indeed, subsequent research has generalised findings initially focused on OECD countries, which concluded that the concentration of incomes at the top impeded growth, whereas growth, in contrast, was stimulated by increasing the portion of total wealth going to the lowest quintile of the population or to the middle class: researchers from the IMF thus found 'an inverse relationship between the income share accruing to the rich (top 20%) and economic growth':

> If the income share of the top 20 percent increases by 1 percentage point, GDP growth is actually 0.08 percentage point *lower* in the following five years, suggesting that the benefits do not trickle down. Instead, a similar increase in the income share of the bottom 20 percent (the poor) is associated with 0.38 percentage point *higher* growth. This positive relationship between disposable income shares and higher growth continues to hold for the second and third quintiles (the middle class). (Dabla-Norris et al, 2015, p 7)

Thus, while low-income countries understandably seek to grow their economies, they can actually do so more effectively by reducing inequality through a combination of progressive taxation and redistribution systems. Strengthening these systems does not hold back these countries: instead, it allows them to move forward, faster.

Yet, despite its benefits (and even, in most cases, its popularity with voters), progressive taxation with powerful inequality-reducing impacts may be difficult to achieve for many governments. Inter-jurisdictional fiscal competition to retain or attract businesses is one factor. Another factor is that indirect taxes (such as VAT) are easier to collect, and therefore, despite their regressive impacts (since poor households spend a higher proportion of their incomes on buying consumer goods [Elson et al, 2013]),[3] they may be the preferred way for governments with a weak administrative capacity to collect revenue. Third, because capital is more mobile than labour and households, it is tempting to reduce the levels of taxation on capital, particularly by lowering the corporate tax and personal income tax for the highest income earners, and to compensate for this by increasing the taxation of wage-earners and households: globally, the top personal income taxes were lowered by about 30% on average since 1980 (International Monetary Fund, 2014, p 37). In any case, taxation is meaningful only when related to social investment: poverty reduction depends not only on how revenue is collected to finance public services and social protection, but also on how public money is spent. It is to this issue that we turn next.

Strengthening social protection: the social investment state

Developing social protection: protecting basic income security

Adequate and effective income support systems, both in cash and in kind, are a key element in combating family and child poverty. Social protection mechanisms such as pensions, fee waivers, child support grants and cash transfers can prevent households from falling into poverty. Such support measures can help households and societies to go through

---

[3]   It is important to note, however, that although VAT is regressive when calculations are made on income (the poorest households contribute more as a proportion of their income), this regressivity either disappears or is significantly attenuated when calculated on the basis of consumption (that is, the higher levels of consumption of the rich and the high VAT rates on luxury items that are affordable only to the rich, leads to a situation in which the rich contribute more to the revenues collected through VAT than do the poor) (see Corbacho et al, 2013, pp 167–168).

economic or climatic shocks. As explained in a UNICEF publication:

> Cash transfers can work as a 'safety net' to keep the poorest, most vulnerable households out of destitution in all settings, including humanitarian emergencies. At the same time, they offer families a ladder out of poverty by boosting incomes, increasing school attendance, improving nutrition, encouraging the use of health services and providing job opportunities. By one estimate, social protection initiatives keep some 150 million people out of poverty, and they make a positive impact on children's lives across a range of indicators. ... Cash transfers work by putting more money into the hands of the poor, strengthening local markets and creating a stream of social benefits that come with poverty reduction. As households spend the transfers they receive, their impact is multiplied in the local economy and the benefits transmitted to others in society. (UNICEF, 2016)

Households supported by cash transfers will be able to afford better healthcare and nutrition for the children. Child labour will decrease, and school enrolment and learning outcomes will improve. Child marriage will be reduced, as early marriage, for girls, is often a means for the family to save money by having one less mouth to feed (Save the Children, 2020a). Programmes such as India's midday-meal scheme or Ethiopia's productive safety net thus have made a measurable impact on children's well-being (Young Lives, 2008). In rural Bangladesh, an initiative to empower girls through conditional incentives for households of adolescent girls led to substantial reductions in child marriage and teenage childbearing in a setting with high rates of underage marriage and had positive effects on educational attainment for girls in school (Buchmann et al, 2018). In South Africa, the introduction of cash transfers had a major impact in reducing the transmission of mental health issues from parents to children (Eyal and Burns, 2016).

Social protection has an equally important role in combating child poverty in high-income countries. In the EU, almost one in four children (22.2%) are at risk of poverty or social exclusion, with lifelong consequences for the child concerned; only 16% of all children under three are in formal childcare; and in more than one third of EU Member States, low-income families find ECEC to be unaffordable (De Schutter, 2021b, paras 37–40). Greater attention has been going to addressing this challenge in the EU. Already in 2013, the EU Recommendation on Investing in Children acknowledged the need to support household incomes through adequate, coherent and efficient benefits, including fiscal incentives, family and child benefits, housing benefits and minimum-income schemes, and to complement cash income-support schemes with in-kind benefits related in particular to nutrition, childcare, education, health, housing, transport and access to sports or socio-cultural activities. It highlighted the importance of adequate redistribution across income groups, ensuring easy take-up, avoiding stigmatisation and ensuring regular and responsive delivery mechanisms (European Commission, 2013). Indeed, the countries with the lowest rates of child poverty or social exclusion are those that provide adequate, coherent and efficient benefits (including through an adequate balance of universal and targeted schemes, by avoiding inactivity traps, by reflecting the evolution of household types and ensuring redistribution across income groups). The most effective systems limit conditionality and thus reduce problems of non-take-up (Frazer and Marlier, 2013). More recently, acting on the basis of a proposal of the European Commission, the Council of the EU adopted the European Child Guarantee, which should ensure that 'children in need' in the EU have effective and free access to ECEC, education (including school-based activities), a healthy meal each school day and healthcare; and effective access to healthy nutrition and adequate housing.[4] And, in January 2023, the Council of the EU adopted a Recommendation on adequate minimum income ensuring active inclusion (Council of the EU, 2023), which 'aims at combatting poverty and social exclusion by promoting adequate income support, in particular by means of minimum income, effective access to enabling and essential services for persons lacking sufficient resources and fostering labour market integration of those who can work, in line with the active inclusion approach'. The recommendation should ensure that EU Member States adopt a 'transparent and robust methodology' to define the adequate level of support 'that guarantee[s] life in dignity at all stages of life, by combining adequate income support – through minimum income benefits and other accompanying monetary benefits and in-kind benefits, and giving access to enabling and essential services'. It includes specific provisions aimed at reducing the rates of non-take-up, to close the gap between legal coverage and effective coverage of minimum-income schemes, by simplifying the administrative procedures and by proactively reaching out to beneficiaries and ensuring they have access to information about their rights.

For most countries, insufficient fiscal space will constitute the major obstacle to the provision of social protection at levels that effectively prevent households from falling into poverty. Countries that are heavily indebted, in particular, may be hesitant to make support to low-income households a priority. Social protection, however, should be seen not as a cost imposing a burden on a country's finances: it should

---

[4] In order to help set a baseline for monitoring the implementation of the European Child Guarantee, the European Commission asked the European Social Policy Analysis Network (ESPAN) to assess the extent to which, in 2023, children at risk of poverty have access to these six services in each of the 27 EU Member States. See Baptista et al (2023).

be seen as an investment, with high returns resulting from its contribution to the inclusive growth of the country. Providing income support to people throughout their lives is therefore not only a human rights obligation – it makes economic sense as well.

There are a number of reasons for this. At household level, social protection allows households to increase their savings, protecting them from having to sell productive assets in times of crisis and from being driven into destitution because of catastrophic health payments (Ralston et al, 2017). More generally, social protection (and minimum-income support in particular) allows households to escape the 'scarcity trap', which may lead them to make choices that are sub-optimal in the long run: where the focus is on the short-term imperative of making ends meet in order to ensure that immediate priorities are met (that rent and electricity bills are paid, and that food is on the table), it may be particularly challenging to escape the 'tunnel' of meeting such immediate needs, and to have enough 'bandwidth' to accommodate other considerations (Mullainathan and Shafir, 2013). At a more macro level, social protection plays a stabilising role in times of economic downturn because of its poverty-alleviation impacts and its ability to raise consumption levels of low-income households: it is thus a powerful counter-cyclical tool.[5] Social protection is also critical to ensure inclusive and sustainable growth, favouring a form of development that is more equally shared, with more significant poverty-reduction impacts (UNDP et al, 2011). In countries such as Brazil, Mexico or Chile, conditional cash transfers reduced inequality levels (measured according to the Gini coefficient) by 21% (for Brazil and Mexico) or 15%

---

[5]　This role of social protection – in smoothing business cycles – was emphasised for instance by the assessment of Ghana's Livelihood Empowerment Against Poverty (LEAP) cash transfer programme, which provides cash and health insurance to extremely poor households for more than 70,000 households across Ghana (Handa et al, 2014).

(Chile) between the mid–1990s and the mid–2000s, although such programmes represent only less than 1% of the GDP (Soares et al, 2007).

Perhaps even more significant if we consider it as an investment, social protection has significant multiplier effects for the local economy, since beneficiaries spend in local businesses. Using the LEWIE (local economy-wide impact evaluation) model to assess multiplier effects of cash transfers across seven sub-Saharan African countries, FAO found that nominal income multipliers range from 2.52 in Ethiopia to 1.34 in Kenya (FAO, 2017). Subsequent research on two cash transfer schemes in Zambia (CGP and Multiple Categorical Targeting Grant) generated income multipliers averaging 1.67 in both programmes (Handa et al, 2018).

And social protection improves competitiveness: it leads to increased school enrolment and success, improved health outcomes and higher labour market participation rates, thus benefiting local economies at large.

Social protection allows families to invest more in the education of children, resulting in the strengthening of what the economic literature calls 'human capital', the expression made popular by the economist Gary Becker (Becker, 1964). For instance, cash transfers reduced child participation on family farms in Kenya, Lesotho, Ethiopia and Zimbabwe (FAO, 2017). In India, child labour was reduced by 13.4% for boys and by 8.2% for girls when the National Rural Employment Guarantee scheme was introduced in 2005 with a commitment to provide a minimum of 100 days per year of labour paid at the minimum wage to rural households (Sanfilippo et al, 2012). Similar results have been registered with the Social Cash Transfer Pilot Programme in Ethiopia, as described in a publication tellingly titled *The Business Case for Social Protection in Africa* (Gassmann et al, 2018). School enrolment rates for girls increased significantly in countries such as Ecuador (Araujo et al, 2017), Lesotho (FAO, 2017) or Pakistan (Sanfilippo et al, 2012). In Latin America, conditional cash transfer programmes have also been found to reduce the probability of school absenteeism and grade repetition, increasing attendance and educational attainment among boys and girls alike: this was confirmed by studies on Paraguay (Veras Soares et al, 2008), Nicaragua (Maluccio and Flores, 2005) and Mexico (Parker and Vogl, 2018), as well as Colombia: evaluation of 'Familias en Acción', a conditional cash transfer programme implemented in rural areas in Colombia since 2002, concluded for instance that the programme increased school participation of 14–17-year-old children by between 5 and 7pp, and also significantly reduced domestic work for children, particularly younger children (although income-generating child work was barely affected) (Attanasio et al, 2010). Similar conclusions were reached for cash transfer schemes in Africa, for instance in Ghana (Handa et al, 2014).

Even old-age pension schemes have these impacts, since the increased disposable income of households is often invested in education. Recipients of the old-age grant in Lesotho spend a substantial proportion of their grant on uniforms, books, and stationery for their grandchildren (Omilola and Kaniki, 2014); the Kalomo programme in Zambia, which benefits households headed by older people, has led to a 16% increase in school attendance (Omilola and Kaniki, 2014).

Nutrition and health outcomes are also significantly improved thanks to social protection. While 'Bolsa Família' in Brazil is perhaps the most-studied example of the contribution of social protection to food and nutrition security (see, for instance, Dest, 2009), many other cases have shown increases in caloric intake, number of meals per day and food production as a result of social assistance schemes. In South Africa and Mexico, old-age pensions and food subsidies have been documented to lead to taller and overall healthier children (Sanfilippo et al, 2012). In India, the National Rural Employment Guarantee Scheme substantially increased participants' caloric and protein intake (Deininger and Liu, 2013). In Ethiopia, the Social Cash Transfer Pilot Programme decreased by 0.24 the number of months in which households suffered from food shortage and increased by

0.6 the number of times children and adults ate per day (Asfaw et al, 2016); and participating households in the Productive Safety Net Programme decreased food shortage by 1.29 months in the dry season, as compared to non-beneficiaries (Berhane et al, 2014). For every dollar transferred to households in African countries, US$0.36 is used on food expenses: improved food security is the first and most immediate impact of the introduction of social protection (Handa et al, 2014).

At the same time, while adequate income support systems for households with children are a key element in combating child malnutrition, a range of other policies can also play an important role in improving nutritional outcomes. In India, for instance, at the end of 2001, a first Supreme Court order directed state governments to provide cooked midday meals in all government primary schools following the so-called 'right to food case'.[6] As explained by Drèze: 'In due course, midday meals came to be seen as one of India's most effective social programmes (a substantial body of research brings out their positive impact on school attendance, child nutrition, and pupil achievements)' (Drèze, 2019, pp 69–70; for useful analysis and evidence on the topic in the same volume, see also *inter alia* the section 'Midday Meals and the Joy of Learning' [pp 81–84]).

In the same spirit, in preparation of the European Child Guarantee, proposals were made regarding a range of policies aimed at improving nutritional outcomes of children: the provision of healthy school meals in primary and secondary schools; educational activities on healthy food, such as school breakfasts that empower children to act as advocates for better nutrition in their families and communities; schemes that can

---

[6] The so-called 'right to food case' (*People's Union for Civil Liberties [PUCL] vs Union of India and Others, Writ Petition [Civil] 196 of 2001*) went on for 16 years. Over time, the case had a bearing on many of the Indian social programmes, especially midday meals, the creation of integrated child development services, and the public distribution system of food grains (mainly rice and wheat). The case also facilitated the growth of a wider campaign for the right to food (Drèze, 2019).

reach children in their home environments, such as food banks or meal-at-home programmes to support households lacking sufficient food; or the promotion of breastfeeding. Food environments can also be transformed in order to encourage healthy eating habits, for instance by introducing 'no fry' zones around schools to limit the availability of high-fat fast food (Bradshaw and Rees, 2019; Frazer et al, 2020).

Beyond food and nutrition security, health outcomes more generally gain from social protection. Paid parental leave has been associated with higher vaccination rates for children (parents face less work-related limitations to vaccinating their children [Daku et al, 2012; Heymann et al, 2017]), with lower infant mortality (Nandi et al, 2016) and with increased rations of breastfeeding (which also contribute to children's immunisation and reduced risks of obesity [Chai et al, 2018]). Children whose parents benefit from social protection are healthier and more productive as adults.

Contrary to a common prejudice, moreover, social protection does not discourage the search for employment.[7] Instead, it often increases labour market participation. Social protection schemes that take the form of asset transfers or public works programmes are particularly effective in encouraging labour market participation. Asset transfers, which take the form, for instance, of the provision of livestock or tools to start a small business combined with some form of training, allow beneficiaries to start a small business of their own, with sometimes remarkable results: this is famously illustrated by the so-called graduation model pioneered by the non-governmental development organisation (BRAC) in Bangladesh (Banerjee et al, 2017). Public works programmes can be designed to improve the level of qualifications of the participants: in Sierra Leone, households benefiting from a

---

[7] Old-age pension constitutes of course an exception in this regard, since its very purpose is to allow people having reached pensionable age to retire without having to continue to work.

public works programme were 34% more likely to have paid work after the project ended (Gassmann et al, 2018), and participant households were four times more likely to invest in new businesses (Rosas and Sabarwal, 2016). Similar results are reported for Egypt and Tunisia (Mvukiyehe, 2018).

Social protection schemes that take the form of cash transfers show more mixed results on employment. In general, the amounts provided are too low to be an incentive not to seek employment (or to move away from employment). One of the earliest and most famous conditional cash transfer programmes is the 'Oportunidades' programme introduced in Mexico in 2002 ('Oportunidades' built on an earlier version called 'Progresa' which started in 1997, and it was later relabelled 'Prospera', before being phased out). Seventeen years after its launch, the programme was assessed for its employment impacts: it was found that the participants in the programme for three years were 13.7pp more likely to be employed, worked 2.9 hours more per week and earned 1.4 pesos more per hour than the comparable non-participant population; moreover, any additional year during which the participants benefited from 'Oportunidades' improved their employment prospects by 4.5pp (Kugler and Rojas, 2018). But other empirical evidence is more ambiguous. In 2019, a team of researchers from the UN's Economic Commission for Latin America and the Caribbean (CEPAL) considered a total of 87 evaluations of 21 conditional cash transfer programmes, covering 13 countries of the region: while the impacts on labour integration (measured, for instance, by participation rate or hours worked) were positive in 53% of the cases, they were negative in another 47% (Abramo et al, 2019, p 68).

The CEPAL study also showed results that were less encouraging for women than for men. This last finding probably simply shows that women face obstacles to labour market participation that are separate from, and additional to, an inability to invest in education and training in order to improve their chances on the labour market. At the same time, the evidence also shows an interesting spill-over effect of cash transfer programmes on the allocation of women's time between work outside the home and household chores or care for the elderly. The single most consistent finding across studies is that cash transfer programmes reduce child labour (Bastagli et al, 2016, p 178). As a result, women may seek waged employment in order to compensate for the loss of earnings for the family owing to the withdrawal of children from the labour market: this was, for instance, a conclusion from an evaluation of 'Familias en Acción', a conditional cash transfer programme in Colombia, which had positive effects on the female labour supply, especially in rural areas (Attanasio and Gómez, 2004).

Some comparative studies conclude that cash transfers can have a positive impact on employment. In order to assess whether such programmes (conditional or not) discouraged labour market participation by working-age adults, a team of researchers relied on randomised controlled trials conducted in three Latin American countries (Honduras, Mexico and Nicaragua), two in Asia (Indonesia and the Philippines) and one in Africa (Morocco) (Banerjee et al, 2017). They concluded that cash transfer programmes, whether conditional or not, do not discourage labour market participation by working-age adults. Whereas, in theory, such programmes could lead individuals to work less, due either to an 'income effect' (the income from the cash transfer programme makes it unnecessary to work), or to the fear of individuals that they will lose certain social benefits if they increase their income from work, in most cases, the positive spill-over effects predominate: beneficiaries of cash transfer programmes more easily start as entrepreneurs or can take up employment more easily due to improved health and training. In their review of 80 impact evaluations of 56 conditional or unconditional cash transfers worldwide (covering a total of 30 low- and middle-income countries for the period 2010–15), Overseas Development Institute researchers also found no reduction in the labour supply attributable to such programmes (Bastagli et al, 2016). Indeed, labour market participation of working-age adults was found in some studies to be positively encouraged by cash transfer programmes. The Brazilian 'Bolsa Escola' school grant programme, for instance, which ran between 2001 and 2003, increased labour market participation by mothers and fathers of programme recipients by around 3pp (Ferro, Kassouf and Levison, 2010). And the other major Brazilian conditional cash transfer programme, 'Bolsa Família', enabled a rise the proportion of people seeking work, especially for women (Camilo de Oliveira et al, 2007; see also Ribas and Soares, 2011).

The evidence of the impacts of cash transfer schemes on participation in the labour market is therefore somewhat mixed but largely positive. The interpretation of such empirical results, however, should take into account the fact that the receipt of social support, as it provides greater income security, strengthens the bargaining power of beneficiaries, who may be in a better position to resist job offers that pay misery wages or provide precarious working conditions. Therefore, at least part of the potentially positive impacts of cash transfers on participation in the labour market may be offset by the fact that these beneficiaries may wait, until they take up employment, for a decent job to be proposed: there is some evidence of this in studies of the impacts of 'Bolsa Família' in Brazil and of the Human Development Grant in Ecuador (Ribas and Soares, 2011; González-Rozada and Llerena, 2011).

In what follows, we summarise the reasons why, within social protection in general, investments in ECEC are particularly crucial to break the cycles perpetuating poverty. We also explore what role schools and healthcare services may play in this regard. Tackling child poverty is crucial, but to address it does not mean the focus should be on the child alone: unless the household's living conditions are improved, the stress of scarcity will continue to leave its mark on the child, creating a significant obstacle to equality of opportunities.

Investing in early childhood

Social protection will be particularly effective in breaking the vicious cycles that perpetuate poverty if they reach children during early childhood. Children born into poverty face major obstacles: it is in that sense that a society which tolerates poverty betrays the ideal of equal opportunities. Yet, these children are not doomed to fail. While the stress experienced by families living in poverty may have long-term impacts on the child through various physiological mechanisms, such impacts can be largely buffered by supportive parenting.

Such supportive parenting in turn can be helped by improved income security. The increase in paid and unpaid maternity leave in Norway in 1977, for instance, led on average to a 2pp decline in high school dropout rates and a 5% increase in wages for the children at age 30, with even more important gains (around 8% higher wages at age 30) when the mothers had lower education levels (Carneiro et al, 2015). Universal child benefits are particularly effective in this regard, since they reduce the risks of under-inclusion and stigmatisation associated with targeting (Save the Children, 2020c).

Interventions during early childhood are the most likely to be effective. As the WHO–UNICEF–Lancet Commission has reported, follow-up studies of children exposed to poverty, from a wide range of countries, show the beneficial effects of early childhood interventions for adult earnings, cognitive and educational achievement, health biomarkers, reductions in violence, reduction of depressive symptoms and social inhibition, and growth (for example, increasing birthweight and head circumference) in the subsequent generation. In Jamaica, two years of psychosocial stimulation to growth-stunted toddlers increased earnings by 25% 20 years later, sufficient to catch up with individuals who were not stunted as children. In the US, the HighScope Perry Preschool programme had estimated annual social rates of return of

7–12% meaning that every dollar invested resulted in US$7–12 benefit per person (The Lancet, 2020). It has often been remarked that the first 1,000 days of a child's life are crucial to a child's development, and are the most formative time for health, growth and cognitive development that set the path for adulthood: these first 1,000 days are therefore the period where the return on investment in children is highest, be it in health, early child development or nutrition, and will allow them to reach their full potential and maximise their contribution to society (Save the Children, 2020b). Support to children and families at risk of poverty or social exclusion and in vulnerable situations when children are at a very early age is therefore one of the keys to preventing barriers developing which hinder children's development. It can help to ensure a positive trajectory which reduces problems of poor health and increases children's ability to participate in education and to access other services (Frazer et al, 2020).

Early childhood interventions face two major obstacles, however. First, even where public programmes supporting low-income households exist, such households, especially those with lone parents, may be poorly informed about such programmes or otherwise unable to claim the support that is available in theory: this phenomenon, referred to as the 'non-take-up of rights' in the social policy literature, affects particularly low-income households with limited access to the internet and social networks, and therefore a limited ability to overcome the many bureaucratic hurdles to access social protection (De Schutter, 2022b). Home visits providing information, resources and support to expecting parents and families with young children may be an important tool to overcome obstacles and reduce rates of non-take-up (Duggan et al, 2018). Home visiting programmes are expensive in the short run, but the positive impacts in the medium and long term are very high, including by improving employment prospects for the children and by reducing the families' need for public assistance programmes (Michalopoulos et al, 2017).

The non-take-up of rights can also be addressed through ensuring that legal entitlements are clear and transparent and are accompanied by outreach and information to parents from vulnerable backgrounds and by simplifying administrative barriers (Frazer et al, 2020). There may be a tension, however, between reducing rates of non-take-up on the one hand and, on the other hand, ensuring that interventions are effectively focused on low-income households that are the most in need of support. In general, targeting implies that access to social protection is made conditional on proving income levels, which typically requires either that the individual claiming a benefit provides documentation about income levels or that social services rely on proxy means testing, where data are collected as a 'proxy' for household income. These methods can have significant exclusionary impacts: documentation may be difficult to collect (or to pay for) for low-income households, and such households, for instance because they live in informal settlements, are routinely left out from social registries (De Schutter, 2022b).

Therefore, a balance may have to be struck (or an adequate combination found) between the benefits of targeting and the advantages of universalistic approaches to the delivery of social protection and social services more generally. The principle of 'progressive' (or 'tailored') universalism (as advocated by Frazer et al, 2020) means that welfare states should be inclusive, and that people at the bottom of the distribution should benefit at the same time as others in society. In practical terms, this approach combines both universal and targeted policies: it suggests that those in need should receive more support than other population segments to compensate for disadvantages. From the perspective of progressive universalism, targeting and mainstream can coexist; they are compatible and, in fact, mutually reinforcing concepts. However, effective progressive universalism for children requires information systems that – during the planning and implementation processes – identify and prioritise the children most in need of additional support.

It also requires the identification of targets to be achieved as well as adequate systems of monitoring and reporting.

There is a second obstacle to the provision of support to low-income households, where such support goes through social services. Well-resourced social services are essential to supporting low-income households (Acquah and Thévenon, 2020; Frazer et al, 2020), particularly at the local level (Montero 2016). Disadvantaged families have often developed considerable suspicion towards such services, however, thus impeding the ability of these services to provide effective support. This is partly due to the fact that social services are increasingly asked to act as gatekeepers to prevent households from abusing the social protection system and to prevent fraud. It is also due to the fact that children living in poverty are particularly at risk of being separated from their families (PACE, 2015; Chaitkin et al, 2017). Under international human rights law, removing a child from the family should be a measure only of last resort: article 9 of the Convention on the Rights of the Child provides that children have the right not to be separated from their biological parents, unless such separation is in their best interests, and the Committee on the Rights of the Child is clear that 'economic reasons cannot be a justification for separating a child from his or her parents' (UN Committee on the Rights of the Child, 2013, para 61). However, institutional actors still occasionally encourage parents to place their children so as to ensure that they will receive food, education, healthcare and shelter (Doyle, 2010, p 5).

This may constitute a strong reason for parents to fear contacts with social services, and it is thus another cause for the non-take-up of rights in the field of social protection. It is therefore essential to invest in professional training to foster an approach that is seen as supportive and transformational rather than controlling, to increase representation of minorities among social workers, to foster a holistic approach built around integrated community services, to emphasise prevention and to promote parental advocacy. Gatekeeping mechanisms should also be put in place to ensure that children are placed in alternative care only if all possible means of keeping them with their parents or extended family have been examined (Lerch and Nordenmark Severinsson, 2019). Improved ECEC and support to disadvantaged families are essential to break the cycles of poverty, and the role of social services in this regard is of course vital. Rather than creating new forms of dependencies, however, the role of social services should be to form partnerships with parents, focused on the best interests of the child, and to promote autonomy of the families through help, parental training and supervision (Council of Europe, 2011). Where there is a risk of abuse, neglect, violence and maltreatment, social services should seek to identify in-home-measures where children can continue living with their families and communities rather than separating and placing them in residential or family-based care. In the exceptional cases where alternative care is deemed necessary and in the child's best interests, it should be ensured that there is a range of alternative care options; that the care placements are taken on a case-by-case basis; and that the period spent in alternative care, and the care received, are suitable to the needs of that individual child. Moreover, when placed into care, children have the right to be in contact with their family if it is in their best interests; international child rights standards call for children under the age of three not to be cared for in residential care under any circumstances.

Promoting inclusive education

There exists a strong relationship between public investments in education and relative mobility, especially for developing economies and regarding primary education (Corak, 2013; Narayan et al, 2018). Investing more in education is therefore essential to break the cycle of poverty. The Education 2030 Framework for Action has set two public education expenditure benchmarks to achieve SDG 4: at least 4% of GDP and at least 15% of total public expenditure. The global trend in education expenditure in 2000–17 was generally flat for both indicators, however, with Latin America and the Caribbean being the exception: while education expenditure as a share of GDP increased in this region from 3.9% in 2000 to 5.6% in 2017 (a high rate compared to the other regions), globally, expenditure as a weighted share of GDP fluctuated around 4.7%, while expenditure as a weighted share of total public expenditure rose only from 12% in 2000 to 12.5% in 2017 (UNESCO, 2020). In OECD countries, the main deficiency concerns early preschool education: while enrolment rates increased significantly between 2005 and 2020 for children between three and five years old, only 27% of children below three years of age have access to early childhood education (OECD, 2022).

Rough indicators concerning access to education are in any case insufficient to correctly assess the challenge of breaking the cycles of poverty. Indeed, schools themselves often cannot fully compensate for differentials in preschool education between disadvantaged and less disadvantaged children, especially where residential segregation between rich and poor is important. More than the resources available to the school or the size of classrooms, what matters is peer influences, teachers' morale and qualifications and the school's emphasis on academic preparation (Putnam, 2015, ch 4).

In other terms, what is needed is a desegregated and inclusive educational system that affirmatively seeks to provide equal opportunities to disadvantaged children. Truly inclusive schools are schools that provide more extracurricular opportunities after school hours (Duncan and Murnane, 2014); that strengthen the links between the school and the community in order to improve social capital and access to various networks for the child; that reduce the role of selection and assessment of children based on academic performance, and instead value each child for what they contribute to the classroom; and that ensure that learning orientations are not biased against low-income children, whose choices and aspirations should be fully respected – rather than ignored or dismissed by the common prejudice that such children cannot succeed in certain study courses that are considered more demanding (ATD Quart Monde and Changement pour l'Egalité, 2017).

Provided that they affirmatively seek to ensure equal opportunities rather than simply reproduce existing inequalities inherited from childhood, schools may provide a second chance to children from families in poverty. More integrated schooling systems also ensure that pupils from wealthier backgrounds will develop a more prosocial behaviour and will be less likely to discriminate against poor students. It diminishes negative stereotyping of the poor, as shown by the branch of social psychology known as the 'intergroup contact theory' (Allport, 1954): Gautam Rao found, for instance, that negative prejudice against poor children diminished after elite schools in Delhi were forced to open more spaces to children from low-income families (Rao, 2019), and a review of 515 studies found that in 94% of the cases, mere intergroup contact (that is, increased diversity) reduced prejudice (Pettigrew and Tropp, 2000).

Important though it is, the removal of financial barriers to accessing education (including the so-called 'hidden costs' linked to the cost of uniforms, of textbooks, of meals or of transport) is thus not enough to create the conditions for a truly inclusive form of education. Some of the key priorities that have been identified in the context of the European Child Guarantee to ensure that children in vulnerable situations have access to inclusive high-quality education include developing equity funding strategies for disadvantaged students in order to equalise educational outcomes through measures such as ensuring smaller class sizes in primary schools in disadvantaged neighbourhoods, channelling additional funds to disadvantaged schools to improve material conditions, transforming disadvantaged/ghetto schools into 'magnet schools' and developing multi-service or extended schools aimed at offering integrated services (covering healthcare, social care, language stimulation, cultural enrichment and psychological support). Various studies have also recommended developing partnership programmes between schools, parents, local communities and social services; developing schools as hubs for the provision of integrated services; and developing all-day schools where children, especially those from economically disadvantaged households, receive free education services (Frazer et al, 2020; Guio et al, 2021).

Investing in inclusive health services

Access to healthcare is essential to maintain a productive workforce and to reduce illness-related absence from work. A range of studies confirm the positive impacts on health resulting from social protection in general, and from improved access to healthcare in particular. In Bangladesh, an impact evaluation of the Ultra Poor Programme showed that recipients were more likely to get immunised, use antenatal and post-natal care, consume vitamin A among children under five years of age and to use modern contraceptive methods (Asian Development Bank, 2012). In Ghana, health insurance and cash transfers increased expenditures on medicines, especially among the extreme poor, that seemed to allocate more resources to medications (Pouw et al, 2017). In Thailand, the Universal Health Coverage programme increased the probability of having annual health check-ups by 9%, with a more significant impact among women (11%); it also increased hospital admission by 2% and outpatient visits by 13% (Ghislandi et al, 2015). In Taiwan, a year after establishing the National Health insurance, previously uninsured older adults increased their use of outpatient care by 15% (Gustafsson–Wright, 2013).

Just as early childhood education is particularly effective in improving educational outcomes, early intervention is crucial to improve health outcomes. In Europe, one of the main conclusions from the Drivers for Health Equity research project on improving health equity through action across the lifecourse, conducted between 2012 and 2015, was that 'providing access to a comprehensive range of quality early years services ... [is essential] to reduce inequalities during the early development of children, especially for those who come from disadvantaged backgrounds'. The research also emphasised the importance of identifying households at risk of poorer health early on, referring them to appropriate services and making special efforts to foster the social inclusion of children who are most vulnerable and at risk of exclusion; and it noted that 'to be delivered effectively, the services should be universal but tailored to social and economic need and recognise parents' knowledge and capacities concerning the development of their children' (Goldblatt et al, 2015). In South Africa the government has recognised that health, and particularly the health of mothers and children, is of particular importance to disrupting the transmission of poverty. They seek to meet this challenge through policies such as the National Integrated Policy for Early Childhood Development, which prioritises essential services such as healthcare, nutrition, social protection, parent support programmes and opportunities for early learning and childcare, targeting primary caregivers and pregnant women (ARC-CRSA, 2016). Another important area to ensure access to quality health services in the context of IGPP is adolescent sexual and reproductive health and rights, access to contraception to unmarried adolescents, targeting also newlyweds (under pressure to conceive).

Indeed, access to adequate healthcare services matters even before birth. Health risks experienced during pregnancy and childbirth can limit children's chances of survival at birth, as well as risk the mother's life. Maternal health is a key determinant of a child's health at birth, not only due to the severe consequences of maternal orphanhood on the child's development (Bird and Higgins, 2011) but also because the deprivations suffered in utero can reduce the effectiveness of post-natal investments (Narayan et al, 2018). Improving maternal health is a key element in improving the health and life chances of children and reducing IGPP.

Investing in decent housing and safe living environments

Another key component of a social investment state is ensuring that all families have access to adequate housing and safe living environments. In Chapter Two, in section 'Housing and living environment', we highlighted how growing up in poor housing and unsafe environments contributes to poverty and social exclusion, and how it also damages children's development, thus contributing to IGPP. Some of the key priorities that have been identified in the context of the European Child Guarantee to ensure that children in vulnerable situations have access to adequate housing and a safe environment include: ensuring that the right to access adequate housing is established in law; developing a comprehensive strategy on access to housing and a strategy for fighting homelessness that gives particular attention to access by children in vulnerable situations and their families to decent-quality affordable housing; increasing the supply of affordable housing and social housing; providing support for utility (water and electricity) bills and mediation mechanisms for managing payment default, as well as debt management; and introducing targeted exemption from house-ownership taxes or council tax as a means for municipal government to reduce financial pressures on owners with children (Frazer et al, 2020). Adequate housing also needs to be accompanied by state investment in measures that create a safe environment for children. Policies are needed to ensure safe drinking water and sanitation, reduce air pollution, end ghettoisation, reduce violence and drugs and foster social networking.

Investing in access to sport, culture and leisure activities

Just as access to ECEC and education are crucial in equipping children to escape poverty, so too is participation in sport, culture and leisure activities but, as was highlighted in Chapter Two, in section 'Impact of poverty on access to sport, culture and leisure activities', children growing up in poverty often lack such opportunities. Sport, culture and leisure activities play a key role through informal education in promoting the well-being and development of both cognitive and non-cognitive skills fostering resilience and effort and broadening social networks, thereby breaking the cycle of disadvantage. The 2013 EU Recommendation on Investing in Children emphasises the importance that such activities play and thus the importance of providing opportunities to participate in informal learning activities that take place outside the home and after regular school hours. To reach children experiencing disadvantage, this requires addressing barriers such as cost, access and cultural differences, providing safe spaces in children's environments and supporting disadvantaged communities by means of specific incentives, encouraging the creation of better after-school activities and enabling all households to participate in social activities that boost parental skills and foster positive family communication (European Commission, 2013).

FIVE

Towards an inclusive economy

Progressive taxation schemes and redistributive social policies, as well as public services such as those discussed already in the fields of education, healthcare, housing, sport and recreation are of course indispensable tools to combat poverty. However, they also present certain limitations. They depend on economic growth, as measured by an increase of the country's GDP per capita. In addition to the ecological barriers that such a strategy now faces, this may create an incentive to create a 'business-friendly' investment climate and to lower the regulatory and tax burdens on corporations, as a means to stimulate wealth creation, with potentially exclusionary impacts: it is a strategy, in other terms, that may encourage the development of an extractive and exclusive economy, when what is needed is a regenerative and inclusive economy. Second, tax-and-transfer approaches may be politically unsustainable, at least where social protection takes the form of welfare policies narrowly targeted to benefit the poor, rather than the middle class: the result of targeting thus conceived is that the median voter may not support such policies, insofar as they are perceived as (and presented by populist politicians as) taking from the rich and deserving groups of the population to provide aid to 'undeserving' poor. It is this finding that is at the heart of the 'paradox of redistribution' highlighted by Korpi and Palme already a generation ago (Korpi and Palme, 1998).

It is therefore vital, in addition to designing progressive taxation schemes and to strengthening social protection and access to essential services, to move towards a more inclusive form of economy, one that ensures real opportunities for all. This is not just a slogan. It means designing a model of development that takes seriously the duty of the state to ensure access to employment. It may require providing social support to young adults, particularly from low-income backgrounds, to compensate for the obstacles they face and reduce the perpetuation of advantage and of disadvantage. It means, finally, taking seriously the prohibition of discrimination on grounds of poverty, in order to combat effectively all forms of povertyism. We consider these tools in turn.

A jobs-rich model of development: making the right to work a reality

Given the negative impact on children's well-being and development of growing up in households with low resources, a key element in breaking the cycle of poverty must be developing a range of policies to enhance access to adequate income and resources for these households. Improving access to employment for adults from low-income backgrounds therefore has an essential role to play in combating child poverty.

How to achieve this? The focus since the 1990s has been on supply-side factors, rather than on the demand side of the employment market; on the individual's incentives to work, rather than on the structural factors that society can influence. The emphasis on ensuring that 'work pays' belongs to that approach, and it is of course essential that in-work poverty be addressed, if it is to provide a remedy against the perpetuation of poverty (see Peña-Casas et al, 2019). Similarly, lifelong learning and training policies can support parents' access to the labour market by ensuring that they acquire the 'right' qualifications: those that the market demands. Finally, the obstacles to employment that result, especially for women, from family responsibilities, can be addressed by promoting family-friendly working conditions (such as parental leave, workplace support and flexible working arrangements); by ensuring access by disadvantaged groups to affordable quality childcare; and by the promotion of gender equality in the labour market and in family responsibilities.

All these tools matter and should be strengthened further. Another approach, however, complementary to the policies that focus on the individual, is to impose on governments a duty to ensure that each individual able and willing to work will be provided with a job, paid at least a living wage and offering working conditions consistent with the requirements of a decent job.

This would go beyond the right to work as it is currently recognised in international human rights law, most notably in article 6 of the International Covenant on Economic, Social and Cultural Rights. Until now, this right has not been interpreted as requiring from states that they provide jobs to the long-term unemployed. Instead, it has been read more narrowly, as imposing on states obligations of means, rather than obligations of result. As expressed in the ILO Employment Policy Convention, 1964 (No 122), states have a duty to adopt 'an active policy designed to promote full, productive and freely chosen employment'. In other terms, states must endeavour to promote employment, by appropriate macroeconomic and fiscal policies; but they are excused if they fail to guarantee a job for all. It is now time to ask whether the interpretation should be revised.

The proponents of the 'Job Guarantee' idea, in particular within the Levy Economics Institute at Bard College (Tcherneva, 2020), take as their departure point that unemployment has huge costs both to the individual and to society. For those affected, unemployment is not only a loss of income, significantly increasing the risk of poverty (Sen 1997). It also results in a depletion of skills and in a loss of confidence for individuals. It exposes to discrimination: employers are reluctant to hire long-term unemployed candidates, since they tend to interpret the fact that a person has been unemployed for long periods of time as betraying a lack of motivation (Van Belle et al, 2018).

In addition to its impact on the individual, unemployment imposes a huge cost on society. It represents a waste of talent, when so many societal needs are still unmet. In advanced economies that provide unemployment benefits or social aid, unemployment has to be compensated for with public funds, to provide basic income security to the individual. In addition to those direct costs, unemployment has a range of indirect costs (Watts and Mitchell, 2000). It is also correlated with poor health and depression, and with higher crime rates (Raphael and Winter-Ebner, 2001). The failure to address unemployment may compound the impacts of an economic crisis, since the decrease in demand may create the conditions for a longer recession. In local communities where layoffs take place, indirect job destruction spreads like a disease to surrounding areas (Tcherneva, 2019).

In contrast to the general acceptance of mass unemployment as a permanent feature of the economy (and, for some, as a convenient means to justify paying workers less), the 'Job Guarantee' recognises that each individual has a right to work (Mitchell, 1998). Its basic premise is that governments, including in particular local government, or private entities with the support of public funding, will provide a decent job at acceptable conditions (including a fair remuneration) to each working-age individual who seeks to work, if that individual is unable to find employment at acceptable conditions elsewhere.

A society that provides a Job Guarantee recognises that each individual has a valuable contribution to make to social progress. It is a society that recognises the worthiness of each of its members, and that refuses the idea that some are redundant. It is also a society that acknowledges the distinction between employment that is created in response to demand, as expressed by the market, and employment that is created in response to societal needs, including needs that the market cannot satisfy because no household or enterprise is willing and able to pay.

Jobs that benefit the local community or society as a whole, rather than only the specific employer, will typically be economically viable only if supported through the public purse. This is the case for jobs that establish or maintain 'commons', such as ecosystems or projects that are accessible to all, from collective vegetable gardens to community-led energy cooperatives, public housing projects and initiatives in the sharing economy; jobs that contribute to the circular economy, encouraging the repair, reuse and recycling of consumer items; and jobs that provide care and support to groups of the population that cannot afford to pay for such support themselves – including older persons, people with disabilities or low-income households. The type of jobs generally proposed in the context of the Job Guarantee are often not prioritised or seen as financially viable by the private sector, which means that most of these jobs do not compete with private sector jobs.

Guaranteeing the right to work through a Job Guarantee can be costly (since the jobs created will be financed by the state). Yet, the immediate fiscal implications should be balanced against the enormous benefits, both for the individual and for society, of combating long-term unemployment. In addition to the savings involved – since unemployment benefits or social aid to the job-seekers can be suspended – the workers provided with employment will spend as consumers and contribute to social insurance schemes. The services they will provide will benefit society, meeting needs that, in the absence of a solvent demand, markets currently cannot respond to, and can contribute to environmental sustainability. This will also give meaning to their work, bringing it closer to what one scholar has described as 'socially capability-enhancing work', in contrast to dominant approaches to labour that value it only to the extent that it is so-called 'productive' work, that is, work valued by the market (Bueno, 2022; Veltman, 2016).

An additional benefit of introducing a Job Guarantee is that it will serve to de-commodify labour – the immediate implication being that, in all the branches of the economy, including in the profit-driven sectors, the bargaining position of workers will be strengthened, since they have the fall-back option of seeking decent employment paid for by the public purse. In 1919, article 427 of the Treaty of Versailles stated that 'labour should not be regarded merely as a commodity or article of commerce', and this principle was again enunciated in 1944, in the ILO Declaration of Philadelphia. It is this idea that the Job Guarantee will help to realise.

Two fears have been expressed in the debate concerning the introduction of a Job Guarantee through public employment schemes. First, it is said, the introduction of the Job Guarantee could be used as a convenient pretext for making social protection conditional on accepting a job, provided such a job is considered 'suitable'. This is a legitimate concern. There exists a strong political pressure to increase work requirements within existing social protection support, a trend sometimes described as the 'activation' of social protection (De Schutter, 2015). In countries where social protection is weak and fiscal space limited, it also may be politically easier to provide income security by establishing or expanding public employment programmes, rather than by expanding other forms of (unconditional) social protection.

The shift 'from welfare to workfare' is not inevitable, however. Participation in the scheme should be on a strictly voluntary basis, not as a condition for receiving other kinds of support. The introduction of a Job Guarantee scheme could be paired with a requirement of non-retrogression in the provision of unconditional social protection, to avoid a slide towards workfare. It could also be combined with initiatives to better value care work, performed within households or communities, often without remuneration or even formal recognition.

Second, some actors, unions in particular, have expressed the fear that public employment programmes could lead to lowering public sector wages, and to weakening the bargaining position of public sector unions, since such programmes would lead to the creation of low-paying jobs to perform the same duties as traditional public sector jobs: public administrations may be tempted to downsize certain services and to outsource them to the Job Guarantee scheme. Yet, this too is not inevitable. Such a consequence would follow only if the wages paid in the Job Guarantee scheme were lower than market wages – for instance if they corresponded to no more than the statutory minimum wage. However, leaving aside the fact that in many developing countries many informal jobs are in fact paid at wages below the minimum wage, the Job Guarantee scheme can be designed to provide better wages and working conditions, thus raising the bar across the employment market and strengthening the bargaining power of workers across the economy (Atkinson, 2015, p 144).

A basic income for young adults

A truly inclusive society, one that is designed to ensure real equality of opportunities, may also rely on the tool of a universal basic income (UBI). While a range of proposals have been made to implement this idea, either to complement classic welfare programmes (Van Parijs and Vanderborght, 2017) or, in a libertarian-conservative version of a 'negative income tax', to replace it (Friedman, 1968), our preferred scenario is that of a UBI introduced to provide all young adults, between the end of secondary education and age 25, with a monthly stipend, on an unconditional basis. This would be providing children from a low-income background with a third chance, where interventions in early childhood and attempts to provide inclusive education remain insufficient. Providing a UBI to support all young adults as they enter into their adult lives may be the most realistic option, both politically and economically: the universal nature of the benefit ensures that it may gain support from large parts of the electorate; and the burden on public budgets would remain bearable, whereas a UBI provided throughout the life cycle, or to all the adult population, could result in difficult trade-offs as other public expenses may have to be cut.

Contrary to a widespread assumption that income support provided unconditionally may discourage work, the provision of a UBI in such a form may in fact favour labour market integration. A study of a randomised cash transfer in Uganda showed that most youth (who normally would not have access to credit in the absence of aid) invested the transfer in vocational skills and tools, leading to significant increases in cash earnings (almost 50% relative to the control group): the real annual return on capital was 35% on average (Blattman et al, 2014). Similarly, an experiment with the introduction of a UBI scheme in rural Kenya shows the benefits of even a relatively modest guaranteed and unconditional income scheme (of the equivalent of US$0.75/day) for improved food security, mental and physical health, and entrepreneurship – protecting households from having to sell productive assets in times of crisis and encouraging them to invest in productive investment (Haushofer and Shapiro, 2016). Studies of UBI schemes in rich countries show either no negative impact on employment or only a marginal impact (a 10% income increase induced by an unconditional cash transfer decreasing labour supply by about 1%), but significant improvements in health and educational outcomes, especially among the most disadvantaged youths (Marinescu, 2018).

By definition, due to its universal nature, UBI for the youth is not stigmatising, and the risks associated with targeting in means–tested programmes are avoided. In most countries, such schemes could be financed by increasing taxes on inheritance. This would also be a coherent way of tackling the growth of wealth inequalities. In OECD countries, the inheritances and gifts reported by the wealthiest households (top 20%) are close to 50 times higher than those reported by the poorest households (bottom 20%), which illustrates the important role of inheritance in perpetuating and even reinforcing inequalities – since wealth inequalities lead to increased income inequalities. Yet only 24 out of 37 OECD countries tax inheritance, estate or gifts across generations, and the levies are typically very low, accounting for only 0.5% of total tax revenues on average for the 24 countries concerned. There are important differences between countries, of course: in the US, only 0.2% of estates are subject to inheritance taxes, and parents may transfer up to US$11 million to their children exempt of taxes, while the figures are 48% and US$17,000 for the Region of Brussels-Capital in Belgium (OECD, 2021a). Overall, however, in combination with the introduction of a UBI scheme for young adults to allow them to pursue their education or to start a small business, taxing inheritance or increasing progressivity in inheritance taxes may be an administratively easy and essentially painless way to break the cycle of poverty. (Thomas Piketty makes a very interesting point in relation to inheritance tax. He suggests that the 'ideal tax system' is 'a compromise between the incentive logic (which favours a tax on the capital stock) and an insurance logic (which favours a tax on the revenue stream stemming from capital)'. He argues that 'the unpredictability of the return on capital explains … why it is more efficient to tax heirs not once and for all, at the moment of inheritance … but throughout their lives, via taxes based on both capital income and the value of the capital stock. In other words, all three types of tax—on inheritance, income, and capital—play useful and complementary roles' [Piketty, 2014, p 527].)

The prohibition of discrimination on grounds of socioeconomic disadvantage

Given the extent to which discrimination causes and perpetuates poverty and social exclusion (see Chapter Two, in section 'Discrimination'), strengthening the protection against discrimination on grounds of poverty (or socioeconomic disadvantage) should be part of any anti-poverty programme. Indeed, under international human rights law, states already have an obligation to address such a form of discrimination. Article 2(2) of the International Covenant on Economic, Social and Cultural Rights mentions 'social origin' and 'property' among the prohibited grounds of discrimination. The Committee on Economic, Social and Cultural Rights has reiterated that people 'must not be arbitrarily treated on account of belonging to a certain economic or social group or strata within society' (UN Committee on Economic, Social and Cultural Rights, 2009, para 35), and it insists that such grounds should be included in the anti-discrimination framework adopted by the states parties to the Covenant.

At its core, the idea is simple enough: people in poverty cannot be treated adversely simply because they are poor; in principle, their underprivileged socioeconomic situation cannot be allowed to result in a reduced ability to enjoy human rights. Yet, discrimination against individuals or groups of individuals on grounds of socioeconomic disadvantage remains widespread, and largely unpunished. The introduction of an explicit protection from discrimination on grounds of social condition in particular would not only have a strong symbolic value, sending a clear message to policy makers in particular that people may not be treated less favourably because they are poor. It would also have institutional consequences, in particular by allowing Equality Bodies (independent institutions tasked with preventing and addressing discrimination and promoting equality) to contribute more effectively to the fight against poverty, alongside the specific contribution other human rights mechanisms can make.

This remains a largely unfinished task. While some progress has been achieved on paper (in the legislative and regulatory framework), the protection from discrimination on grounds of social status is in practice, at best, highly uneven (Thornton, 2018); there are in fact few examples of this ground being used effectively. The European Network of Equality Bodies notes that relying on such a ground of discrimination raises specific challenges, both because 'the meaning, situation and character of the socio-economic status ground is not understood by many people in the society and even within the equality body' and because, in the large majority of cases, discrimination on grounds of social condition (or socioeconomic status) is combined with discrimination on other grounds (particularly sex, race or ethnic origin, disability or age), requiring specific methodologies to be developed to address multiple discrimination appropriately (Equinet, 2010). However, as the Equality Bodies also note, the inclusion of such a ground in anti-discrimination legislation has an essential role to play, not least since poverty is often an obstacle to the filing of discrimination claims, a barrier that the explicit reference to social condition (or socioeconomic status) in the mandate of Equality Bodies could help to overcome – since it would provide a clear encouragement to people in poverty to use the tool of filing individual complaints to challenge discriminatory practices.

The potential role of the prohibition of discrimination on grounds of 'social condition' could be maximised by relying on an expanded notion of the concept of 'social origin' which appears in Article 2(2) of the International Covenant on Economic, Social and Cultural Rights. The Committee on Economic, Social and Cultural Rights (CESCR) understands this expression to refer to the 'social and economic situation when living in poverty or being homeless' (UN Committee on Economic, Social and Cultural Rights, 2009, para 35). As noted by Angelo Capuano, however, this definition may be unnecessarily restrictive, and thus potentially irrelevant in many contexts where discriminatory treatment is based. First, the 'social status' of a person 'is reflected more by prestige and esteem rather than merely property status, wealth or economic status' (Capuano, 2017, p 105). Moreover, 'the criteria which the CESCR seems to use to give content to the concept of "social status" – property status, caste, and economic and social status such as homelessness and poverty – are not likely to be bases upon which an employer will commonly have the opportunity to discriminate' (Capuano, 2017, p 106). Instead, he suggests, discrimination most frequently occurs on the basis of family relationships, of the schools the person has attended or of childhood circumstances: these are instances of 'ascribed status', rather than 'achieved status', and it is these instances in particular that, in such a context, one should be devoting more attention to (Capuano, 2017, pp 109–110).

Two implications follow. A first implication is that, in the understanding of 'disadvantaged socio-economic condition' or simply 'poverty' (whatever the anti-discrimination framework provides for), attention should be paid to both objective and subjective factors – in other terms, to both the circumstances a person faces and the stereotypes or prejudice associated with such circumstances. Guidance may be found in the interpretation provided to the prohibition of discrimination based on the term 'social condition', which appears in Article 10 of the Charter of Human Rights and Freedoms of the Canadian Province of Québec:

> The definition of 'social condition' contains an objective component. A person's standing in society is often determined by his or her occupation, income or education level, or family background. It also has a subjective component, associated with the perceptions that are drawn from these various objective points of reference. A plaintiff need not prove that all of these factors influenced the decision to exclude. It will, however, be necessary to show that as a result of one or more of these factors, the plaintiff can be regarded as part of a socially identifiable group and that it is in this context that the discrimination occurred. (*Comm. des droits de la personne v. Gauthier* [1993], 19 C.H.R.R.D/ 312 [English summary])

A second implication is that, in addition to direct discrimination on grounds of socioeconomic disadvantage or poverty, *indirect* discrimination should be prohibited, where decisions made on other grounds, including on apparently neutral grounds, disproportionately affect people in poverty. Homelessness, for instance, as a proxy for poverty, should not be allowed to lead to discrimination (Farha, 2015, para 39). Employers should not be allowed to reject job applicants based on where they live (in poor neighbourhoods) or on the reputation of the schools the candidate attended (disproportionately attended by pupils from disadvantaged backgrounds). Landlords should not be allowed to refuse to rent an apartment to a lessee who relies on social aid. Schools should not be allowed to penalise students who cannot buy teaching materials or who lack access to the internet. Beyond the diversity of such instances of discrimination, what unites them is that people in poverty are penalised for being poor, adding to the disadvantage that stems from lack of income alone.

Legal tools can be designed to address these situations in their variety. In Ireland for instance, the Equality (Miscellaneous Provisions) Bill 2021 (which is still pending adoption at the time of writing) defines having a socioeconomic disadvantage as being member of a

> socially or geographically identifiable group that suffers from such disadvantage resulting from one or more of the following circumstances: (a) poverty, (b) source of income, (c) illiteracy, (d) level of education, (e) address, type of housing or homelessness, (f) employment status, (g) social or regional accent, or from any other similar circumstance. (Houses of the Oireachtas [Ireland], 2021)

In South Africa, the Promotion of Equality and Prevention of Unfair Discrimination Act (implementing Section 9 of the Constitution) contains a 'Directive Principle' that requires giving special consideration to the inclusion of, *inter alia*, 'socio-economic status' in the list of prohibited grounds: this expression is defined as the 'social or economic condition or perceived condition of a person who is disadvantaged by poverty, low employment status or lack of or low-level educational qualifications'. The formulae may be different, but the central idea remains the same: it should not be allowed to circumvent the prohibition to discriminate on grounds of poverty by using proxies such as a lack of a fixed address, a long-term unemployed status or reliance on social aid, whether such characteristics are relied upon consciously or unconsciously by decision makers.

Public entities, moreover, should not be allowed to make policy decisions or decide regulatory reforms without inquiring into the impacts on people in poverty and ensuring that their decisions do not worsen inequalities. We detail this positive duty further below.[1]

The three roles of equality and non-discrimination in combating poverty

The prohibition of discrimination on grounds of social origin or property extends to any action or omission that disproportionately affects members of a particular group, in the absence of a reasonable and objective justification. (Such form of discrimination is referred to as *de facto* discrimination, to distinguish it from discrimination that is *de jure*, in other terms, that relies explicitly on poverty or socioeconomic condition as a characteristic on which adverse treatment is based.) There is both a negative and a positive face to this. First, regulatory or policy measures that are neutral on their face may be considered discriminatory if they do not take into account the disparate impacts they may have on certain groups of the population, defined for instance on the basis of 'property', or income levels. In South Africa for instance,

---

[1]   See www.legislation.gov.uk/sdsi/2018/9780111038086/body

a Western Cape Equality Court considered that the drastic difference in resources allocated by the South African Police Services to impoverished, predominantly Black communities in comparison to wealthier, White communities amounted to discrimination on the basis of race and poverty, the latter being an 'analogous unlisted ground' on which a claim of discrimination can be based because it 'adversely affects the equal enjoyment of a person's rights and freedom in a serious manner that is comparable to discrimination on a listed ground' (Western Cape High Court, *Social Justice Coalition v Minister of Police*, 2018 ZAWCHC 181, para 65).

It is this idea that is at the heart of a 'positive duty' to consider the impacts on poverty in law and policy making, as imposed for instance in Scotland since April 2018 as part of the Equality Act 2010: this duty, referred to as the 'Fairer Scotland Duty', imposes on a number of public bodies in Scotland to 'actively consider ("pay due regard" to) how they can reduce inequalities of outcome caused by socio-economic disadvantage, when making strategic decisions'.[2] In practice, this means that decisions such as where to locate a school or a hospital, or how to develop a neighbourhood, should be made with the involvement of the local community, and aim at adopting a decision that will reduce, rather than increase, the exclusionary impacts of lack of income – thus contributing to a more inclusive, less divided society. Diana Skelton, a volunteer for ATD Fourth World, described to one of us[3] how low-income families expressed their concerns after plans were announced for the Monklands University Hospital in North Lanarkshire to move: these families were living in the vicinity of the existing hospital, and they feared that they might not be

---

[2] See *Fairer Scotland Duty: Interim Guidance For Public Bodies* (Scottish Government, March 2018), p 5.

[3] At a meeting attended in London by Olivier De Schutter, in November 2019.

able to travel to the new location to seek treatment. Thanks to the consultations that took place, a compromise could be found, providing for some primary healthcare services to remain in Monklands.

Human rights impact assessments serve to alert policy makers to the impacts on the human rights of the poor of the policies they design and implement. Human rights impact assessments, it should be emphasised, are distinct from other types of assessments, including social impact assessments or sustainability impact assessments, with which they present certain similarities. The specificity of human rights impact assessments is that they examine the intended and unintended impacts of policy measures on the ability of the states parties to these agreements to respect, protect and fulfil the human rights of people living in poverty. They therefore should be based explicitly on the normative content of human rights, as clarified by the judicial and non-judicial bodies that are tasked with monitoring compliance with human rights obligations. References in impact assessments to development goals or to poverty are therefore not a substitute for a reference to the normative components of human rights.

The requirement of non-discrimination against the poor is especially important where states face an economic or financial crisis and adopt fiscal consolidation (so-called 'austerity') programmes in order to reassure their creditors as to the health of their public budgets (Bohoslavsky, 2018). In his Letter of 16 May 2012 to the States Parties to the International Covenant on Economic, Social and Cultural Rights on austerity measures, the Chairperson of the CESCR – the expert body tasked with supervising implementation of the covenant – emphasised that fiscal consolidation policies 'must not be discriminatory and must comprise all possible measures, including tax measures, to support social transfers to mitigate inequalities that can grow in times of crisis and to ensure that the rights of the disadvantaged and marginalised individuals and groups are not disproportionately affected'. In a statement adopted in 2016 by the same Committee, it noted, by reference to Article 2, para 2 of the Covenant, that 'Low-income families, especially with children, and the workers with the lowest qualifications are disproportionately affected by measures such as loss of jobs, freezing of the minimum wage and cutbacks in social assistance benefits, potentially resulting in discrimination on grounds of social origin or property' (UN Committee on Economic, Social and Cultural Rights, 2016, para 2). The 2012 Guiding Principles on Extreme Poverty and Human Rights also emphasise this duty, noting that:

> Given the disproportionate and devastating effect of economic and financial crises on groups most vulnerable to poverty, States must be particularly careful to ensure that crisis recovery measures, including cuts in public expenditure, do not deny or infringe those groups' human rights. Measures must be comprehensive and non-discriminatory. They must ensure sustainable finance for social protection systems to mitigate inequalities and to make certain that the rights of disadvantaged and marginalised individuals and groups are not disproportionately affected. (OHCHR, 2012, para 54)

The Guiding Principles on human rights impact assessments of economic reforms presented in 2018 by the Independent Expert on foreign debt and human rights provide further guidance as to how the human rights impacts of fiscal consolidation programmes, as they are adopted following an economic crisis leading to an increase in the sovereign debt and thus additional borrowing by states, should be conducted (Bohoslavsky, 2018).

The equality requirement goes beyond this negative duty, however. In order to prevent discriminatory results, states may have to provide *positively* for differential treatment benefiting certain categories of the population facing systemic disadvantage. In cases of entrenched discrimination, states may be under an obligation to adopt special measures to attenuate or suppress conditions that perpetuate discrimination. Such measures are legitimate under human rights law to the extent that they represent reasonable, objective and proportionate means to redress *de facto* discrimination and are discontinued when substantive equality has been sustainably achieved. Courts have sometimes considered with suspicion differential treatment benefiting certain underprivileged groups defined by their ethnicity or gender – a suspicion which reflects adherence to a formal understanding of equality, resulting in a restrictive reading of non-discrimination law as forbidding the 'sin' of discrimination rather than as a tool to remedy injustices that have their source in society-wide mechanisms of exclusion (Sullivan, 1986). But courts have been far more open to affirmative action measures taken to improve the situation of those who are economically deprived, since socioeconomic condition is not a suspect ground: in fact, such measures are at the very heart of the construction of welfare states, the main purpose of which is to provide support to those who are excluded by the mechanisms of the market.[4]

States therefore should dedicate greater resources to improve the condition of groups who face systemic discrimination (UN Committee on Economic, Social and Cultural Rights, 2009, para 39). They also should move up the causality chain, to tackle the underlying causes of social exclusion. Indeed, once it is recognised that 'a great deal of poverty originates from discriminatory practices – both overt and covert', it follows that poverty-reduction strategies will be fully effective only if they also address 'the socio-cultural and political-legal institutions which sustain the structures of discrimination', and eliminate 'the laws and institutions which foster discrimination against

---

[4] This should be nuanced, since not all welfare states seek to achieve equality: some models aim only at protecting individuals from extreme deprivation, without setting wealth redistribution as an objective in its own right. See Gosta Esping-Andersen (1990).

specific individuals and groups' (OHCHR, 2005, para 21). The fight against inequalities, based in particular on social condition, should concern not only the sphere of economic, social and cultural rights but also the sphere of civil and political rights, since inequalities in access to political influence and socioeconomic inequalities are mutually reinforcing (Alston, 2015, para 21).

Finally, in order to properly assess the contribution of prohibiting discrimination on grounds of socioeconomic disadvantage to breaking the cycles perpetuating poverty, the discrimination faced by disadvantaged individuals and households should be seen for what it is: a form of systemic discrimination which affects a range of areas including health, education, housing and employment.

Addressing discrimination on grounds of socioeconomic disadvantage is therefore ineffective if limited to one sphere alone. For instance, ensuring that employers do not discriminate on grounds of poverty will have a limited impact if disadvantaged individuals continue to face obstacles in having access to quality education, or live in poor neighbourhoods distant from the place of work; supporting schools with a high proportion of disadvantaged pupils may not make a significant difference to these pupils if residential segregation remains unchallenged, so that these pupils remain concentrated in certain schools; and neither combating discrimination in employment nor in education will suffice if health inequalities persist, lowering workers' productivity and academic achievement.

This also points to the limits of an approach to equality of opportunities which relies on classic understandings of 'merit'. In fact, societal improvements pursued in the name of 'meritocracy', including the use of a classic anti-discrimination framework simply prohibiting discrimination but without including class-based affirmative action, could be counter-productive. As emphasised by the Harvard political philosopher Michael Sandel, the more a society promotes meritocracy by insisting on equality of opportunity at the *starting line*, the more it risks justifying whatever inequalities *follow* as the legitimate result of inevitable differences in talent between individuals, combined with the hard work, persistence and discipline of those who succeed (Sandel, 2020). It is not mere coincidence that the belief in meritocracy is entertained in particular by the wealthiest groups within the population (Roex et al, 2019): high-income earners have an interest in believing (and in making believe) that people in poverty are less 'meritorious' and more deserving of their socioeconomic situation, thereby justifying inequality on the basis of unequal merit (Redmond et al, 2002; Heiserman and Simpson, 2017). This is equivalent to blaming people in poverty for being poor, triggering feelings of shame among the poor (Walker, 2014, pp 132–156). Pushed to its limit, 'meritocracy' as an ideology, despite its popularity in public discourse, thus both may reduce empathy towards affected groups and make inequality look like an inevitable and, to some extent, even desirable phenomenon – a means to incentivise people to achieve more. Social psychologists have shown how ideological frames could distort our attentiveness to inequality, and thus our willingness as a society to address it (Waldfogel et al, 2021): this selectiveness towards inequalities (denounced as a scandal where it is based on ethnicity or sex, but seen as legitimate and even desirable where it is seen as attributable to the individual's choices and attitudes) may be one high price to pay for the adherence to a meritocratic ideal of society.

But the meritocratic ideal is problematic at an even more basic level. Reliance on 'meritocracy' is entirely inappropriate, indeed, where disadvantaged individuals have not been given fair opportunities to acquire certain qualifications or to have their experiential competences formally recognised. Instead, affirmative action policies are essential to break the vicious cycles that result from the systemic nature of the discrimination faced by people in poverty. Whereas preferential treatment is well established as regards the allocation of goods or services that *compensate* for poverty or social exclusion, as in means-tested social protection schemes or in the award of scholarships to help overcome financial barriers to education, it is less common and more heavily contested where it is seen to challenge the mainstream narrative about 'deservingness', as in access to employment or to the most coveted schools or universities. Yet, affirmative action is especially needed in such fields, if real equality of opportunities is to be achieved (De Schutter, 2022a, paras 37–40).

Examples abound. Israel successfully designed a form of class-based affirmative action to access the country's most prestigious universities since the mid-2000s, which determines socioeconomic disadvantage on the basis not only of financial status but also of neighbourhood and high school attended, family socioeconomic status (including parental education and family size) and 'individual and/or family adverse circumstances' (Alon and Malamud, 2014). In India, while the Constitution includes various anti-discrimination provisions and bans the practice of 'untouchability' (Art 17), it also states that special measures may be adopted 'for the advancement of any socially and educationally backward classes of citizens', as a means to reduce social inequalities for members of these groups (Art 15, (4) and (5)). This mainly takes the form of reserved seats in public offices and educational institutions (both public and private), as well as job reservations in the public sector, for the castes and tribes mentioned in Articles 341 and 342. In addition however, Article 16(4) of the Constitution allows for 'the reservation of appointments or posts in favour of any backward class of citizens which, in the opinion of the State, is not adequately represented in the services under the State': consistent with this constitutional mandate, the Central Educational Institutions (Reservations in Admissions) Amendment Bill stipulates that 27% of seats are reserved for 'Other Backward Classes' in publicly funded higher education institutions, a policy which led to significant improvement in the socioeconomic diversity in universities (Basant and Sen, 2020).

Affirmative action is in principle acceptable under international law (Bossuyt, 2002). Human rights bodies recognise that it may be required to combat systemic discrimination, and legislation implementing affirmative action programmes occasionally frames such programmes not as a derogation from the principle of equal treatment, but instead as a consequence of that principle. Domestic courts have correctly taken the view that such policies are not a derogation to the principle of non-discrimination, but rather should be seen as implementing the mandate to ensure effective equality, in particular for low-income groups. In *Society for Un-aided Private Schools of Rajasthan v Union of India*, the Indian Supreme Court upheld a requirement imposed on private unaided schools under Section 12(1)(c) of the 2009 Right to Education Act to fill 25% of the seats in Class I with children from weaker and disadvantaged groups, taking into account that the Act sought to remove 'financial and psychological barriers which a child belonging to the weaker section and disadvantaged group has to face while seeking admission', and that this objective could justify reasonable restrictions to the economic freedoms of educational establishments. In Kenya, the High Court allowed a government policy providing more opportunities in national schools to students from public institutions as opposed to students from private institutions: it found that this measure was aimed at achieving substantive equality by reducing the inequality gap between the rich and the poor and was consistent with Article 27(6) of the Kenyan Constitution, which commits the State to give full effect to the realisation of the right to equality and freedom from discrimination by taking legislative and other measures, including affirmative action programmes and policies designed to redress any disadvantage suffered by individuals or groups because of past discrimination.

Affirmative action contributes to increased diversity in different sectors and levels of the professional sphere, providing role models to adolescents and young adults from underprivileged backgrounds. We have also seen how such promotion of diversity can breed greater tolerance and understanding between social groups. Greater diversity also results in decisions made in institutions being better informed by the lived experiences of people in poverty, reducing the risk of indirect (including unconscious) discrimination; and the services provided by such institutions will be more attentive to the specific circumstances of low-income people. Beyond its role as a social-engineering tool, affirmative action recognises the specific obstacles that people in poverty face owing to the persistence of povertyism, thus questioning the mainstream narrative about society distributing outcomes on the basis of 'merit'. This is not merely of symbolic value: it sends a powerful message across society, contradicting the mainstream view about success or failure being attributable to the individual rather than to society's being insufficiently inclusive.

SIX

Making it happen

We know the reasons for IGPP (see Chapter Two) and why breaking the vicious cycles that perpetuate poverty is important not only to low-income households but also to us all (see Chapter Three). We also know that this is possible and what mix of policies and programmes will be needed (see Chapters Four and Five). The challenge we face is to make this happen. The scale of economic, social and environmental changes required, essential though they are for all our futures, will not be easily achieved. It will require placing the goal of ending IGPP at the heart of our economic and political systems and thus in our economic, social and environmental policies. To ensure this will require: raising public and political awareness of and support for tackling IGPP and challenging and debunking some of the myths and prejudices about people living in poverty that can be an excuse for inaction; developing comprehensive and multidimensional strategies which combine universal and targeted policies; putting children's rights at the heart of strategies so as to ensure that no child or person in poverty is left behind; developing better research to inform these strategies; putting in place effective and regular monitoring that will increase accountability for delivering strategies; ensuring that policies and programmes are delivered at local level in an

integrated and holistic way; empowering those living in poverty
to participate in the development and delivery of policies to
end IGPP; and developing stronger links and cooperation
between the poverty and environment agendas.

How to make change happen:

- Invest in raising public and political awareness of and commitment to
  combating IGPP
- Develop comprehensive, multidimensional strategies
- Promote integrated and holistic delivery of policies and programmes at
  local level
- Combine universal and targeted policies – promote progressive universalism
- Count every child and leave no one behind
- Put children's rights at the heart of strategies
- Promote child mainstreaming
- Improve research and data collection
- Enhance monitoring and reporting and increase accountability
- Ensure adequate participation of children and families experiencing
  poverty and social exclusion
- Foster stronger links between the poverty and environment agendas

Investing in raising public and political awareness and commitment to combating IGPP

In developing effective approaches to combatting IGPP and
tackling child poverty it will be important first to raise public
and political awareness of both the positive benefits for children
and society of tackling IGPP and the costs of not doing so.
No one action will do this. Rather, a combination of moral
and utilitarian arguments and evidence will be needed to build
political will and to counter myths and stereotypes about people
in poverty that lead them to be blamed for their poverty and
which are too often used as an excuse for inaction.[1] Combating

---

[1]   Ten myths and stereotypes that often act as blocks to tackling child poverty
and how to respond to them are succinctly explained in a chapter 'Myth

child poverty and reducing inequality should be seen as part of building more social cohesion and more resilient societies. It is also a requirement based on children's fundamental rights. It fosters the well-being of children and their families. It strengthens democracies and increases their credibility. It makes economies more resilient. It is cost-effective. Finally, it is good for social and environmental sustainability. This awareness should then be turned into a clear national commitment to end child poverty, reduce inequalities and thus combat IGPP. Ideally, targets and time-scales for reducing IGPP should be set at country and regional levels as the EU has done (see later, 'Improving research'). The setting of targets requires measuring progress in achieving them. This raises public and political awareness, improves accountability and increases the political costs of inaction. It also fosters debate on policy and programmatic solutions, and thereby increases pressure to gradually improve policies that fail to deliver results (UNICEF and the Global Coalition to End Child Poverty, 2017).

Developing comprehensive, multidimensional strategies

A study on micro and macro drivers of child deprivation[2] in EU countries highlighted that, once household characteristics are taken into account, the provision of public services and affordable education significantly reduces child deprivation, as it can reduce the costs faced by parents; it should be done in addition to the provision of in-cash transfers, which operates through household income (Guio et al, 2022). Various studies have highlighted the key importance of adequate in-cash social transfers and minimum-income schemes to fight against child

---

Buster: Challenging the Stereotypes!' in a 2013 explainer on child poverty (Eurochild and EAPN, 2013, pp 31–40).

[2] At the EU level, child deprivation is defined as the enforced lack of at least three items out of a list of 17 items (including shoes, clothes, food, games, books, celebrations, internet, holidays and so on), see Guio et al (2018).

deprivation (Chzhen and Bradshaw, 2012; Chzhen, 2014; Bárcena-Martín et al, 2017). Across the EU, the countries with the lowest rates of child poverty and social exclusion are generally those which have the most comprehensive packages of inclusive children's policies and programmes reaching out to children from disadvantaged backgrounds (Frazer and Marlier, 2013 and 2017; Frazer et al, 2020; Guio et al, 2021).

This highlights the need for countries to develop integrated packages of policies and programmes to tackle IGPP and child poverty that combine employment policies, cash support and access to services. A multidimensional and integrated approach is needed which covers adequate income, access to good-quality essential services, the participation of children in sport, recreation and cultural activities and the involvement of children and their families in the decisions that affect them. Such an approach has been well set out by the OECD, who stress that 'policy action for disadvantaged children should be coordinated and coherent. The breadth and depth of social inequalities in child well-being mean that efforts are needed in multiple policy areas stretching across multiple government departments and agencies, as well as from other actors inside and outside government' (Clarke and Thévenon, 2022). It has also been highlighted in the work on child poverty in the EU under the Social Open Method of Coordination (Frazer et al, 2010). It is also strongly advocated by a wide range of EU civil society organisations working with children (UNICEF and the Global Coalition to End Child Poverty, 2017; EU Alliance for investing in children, 2020a) and is evident in academic reports.

More recently, the 2021 EU Recommendation establishing a European Child Guarantee specifically recommends EU Member States 'to build an integrated and enabling policy framework to address social exclusion of children, focusing on breaking intergenerational cycles of poverty and disadvantage and reducing the socioeconomic impact of the COVID-19 pandemic'. It recommends that in implementing the Guarantee Member States should 'ensure consistency of social, education, health, nutrition and housing policies at national, regional and local level and, wherever possible, improve their relevance for supporting children in an integrated manner'. In doing this, it requires Member States to develop National Action Plans covering the period to 2030. These plans should include in particular: targeted categories of 'children in need' to be reached by corresponding integrated measures; quantitative and qualitative targets to be achieved in terms of children in need to be reached by corresponding measures, taking into account regional and local disparities; measures planned or taken in implementing this Recommendation (including at regional and local level) and the necessary financial resources and timelines; other measures planned or taken to address child social exclusion and to break inter-generational cycles of disadvantage, based in particular on enabling the policy framework provided; and a national framework for data collection, monitoring and evaluation (Council of the EU, 2021; see also Frazer et al, 2020; European Commission, 2017 and 2021a; Guio et al, 2021).

Promoting integrated delivery of policies and programmes at local level

Setting up a comprehensive and multidimensional strategy will not suffice, however. It is also important to ensure that policies and programmes are delivered in a coordinated, integrated and flexible way at local level. This is important, as people living in poverty often experience a complex set of disadvantages that reinforce each other. These need to be responded to in a holistic manner tailored to the needs of each individual, and not in a piecemeal and haphazard way. Integrated forms of service delivery are therefore often the most effective way of reaching vulnerable families with the highest service needs. This requires improving coordination between different levels of governance and embedding integrated services delivery at the local level – that is, a 'whole system approach' (OECD, 2015b, p 21). This has been reinforced in a subsequent report on the role of family services which emphasises: (i) at government level, the need to foster collaboration between different government bodies, and to ensure adequate funding for early intervention and preventative services; and (ii) at service delivery level, the need to get a better integration between delivery organisations, to build capacities to adapt evidence-based interventions, to share tools to facilitate service implementation, to train practitioners with the necessary skills, to ensure that service delivery fits within the local context and to engage families in services (Acquah and Thévenon, 2020).

Evidence across the EU also shows that countries that tend to do best in combating child poverty and social exclusion encourage an integrated approach so that services reinforce each other, with policies and programmes delivered in an integrated way at local level (Frazer et al, 2020). This highlights the importance of enhancing inter-agency coordination, improving synergies and integration between different policy areas and services for children and improving coordination at and between all levels of governance.

When agencies are open to pooling or sharing their budgets (i.e. the financial resources available to them), this flexibility can facilitate the development of an integrated approach. It is also important that services at a local level adopt child-centred approaches and reach out to the most disadvantaged children and households, emphasise early intervention and promote the empowerment and involvement of children, parents and local communities through a community-development approach (Frazer et al, 2020; Council of the EU, 2021). When developing an integrated approach, it is important to include counselling services and respite services, given that poverty exposes families to high levels of stress.

Combining universal and targeted policies

Effective strategies to tackle child poverty and reduce IGPP need to combine universal policies with additional policies targeted at children and households in vulnerable situations. As we have seen, this is referred to as 'progressive' or 'tailored' universalism. Access to essential services and income security should be ensured for children and low-income households through a combination of two approaches. First, every effort needs to be made to ensure that universal transfers and services for all children are developed in as inclusive a way as possible. This is essential to addressing inequalities between children, to ensure that all children have a decent standard of living and to ensure that children in vulnerable situations have access to the same quality of services and the same opportunities as other children. Good-quality universal public services play a key role in ensuring that all children have access to safety, opportunity and participation. They also avoid the risk that services targeted only at the poor become poor services, and it can be easier to build political support for such services and transfers. Second, to enable some children and their families to access universal services and to receive adequate in-cash transfers, specific additional or complementary policies are needed to meet their specific needs. Such specific policies, by building a bridge towards the mainstream services, should be seen not as an alternative to accessing mainstream provision but as complementary and enabling (Frazer et al, 2020). This is likely to be especially important, when trying to break the cycle of poverty and level the playing field for those children and households experiencing IGPP, to move towards real equality of opportunities.

One reason why such tailored universalism should be prioritised above targeted interventions focused on low-income households alone is that such an approach could free up more public resources for such programmes. The links between universalism/targeting, social spending and redistribution are complex and have been at the heart of a lively debate in social sciences for more than two decades. This starts with what Walter Korpi and Joakim Palme famously described in 1998 as the 'paradox of redistribution': the more countries target welfare resources exclusively at the poor, the less redistribution is actually achieved and the less income inequality and poverty are reduced, because the pro-poor policies will be less politically popular and therefore constitute a low budgetary priority (Korpi and Palme, 1998). In a 2019 state-of-the-art review of the evidence on Korpi and Palme's paradox, Gugushvili and Laenen conclude that 'the only assumption that is unequivocally supported by more recent studies is that higher welfare spending is associated with lower poverty and inequality, but even in this regard there is some indication that countries can compensate for lower spending by more accurate targeting of low-income families'. They go on to state that

> while any general recommendation risks the fallacy of one-size-fits-all, it seems reasonable to suggest that an optimal anti-poverty strategy should contain selective measures alongside more universal programmes. The required balance between the two will inevitably vary across countries, but it seems important that selective policies are not too narrowly targeted at the very poor. Instead, they should also include low-income groups; especially those viewed as more deserving, either because they lack control over their situation (for example, children), or because they pay back society in some way (for example, people who work in low-paid jobs). (Gugushvili and Laenen, 2019, p 120)

Redistribution is influenced by political institutions, ethnic heterogeneity and beliefs about the nature of poverty. The unwillingness of the middle class to support poverty-reduction programmes has been shown to be especially significant where there is a strong correlation between ethnicity and poverty, as in the US or South Africa. Indeed, this is one of the reasons researchers have identified for the differing strength of the welfare state in Europe and in the US: Americans appear to be less willing than Europeans to redistribute from the rich to the poor, in part because poverty in the US largely intersects with 'race' (affecting particularly the African-American community) (Alesina and Glaeser, 2004).

Counting every child and leaving no one behind

There is always a risk with policies to tackle poverty that they focus mainly on those who are easiest to help and that those in the most vulnerable situations are left behind. This is one reason why the SDGs include a commitment to 'leave no one behind' and endeavour 'to reach the furthest behind first' (United Nations, 2015). This will ensure that those experiencing IGPP will be prioritised. A key first step in this regard is to ensure that every child is registered: as the slogan has it, it is not possible to make every child count until every child is counted. This is not of anecdotal importance. Only 45% of children are registered at birth in sub-Saharan Africa, and the same phenomenon plagues other regions: in Bangladesh, only roughly half (56%) of the population is registered (De Schutter, 2021a, para 33). Households in poverty are most affected; for example, among the poorest 30% of households in Indonesia, 71% of children aged under one year did not have a birth certificate in 2012–13, and 88% of adults over 18 years remained unregistered (Sumner and Kusumaningrum, 2015). Thus, a vicious cycle emerges in which the lack of registration of children in poverty results in depriving these children of access to health and education, or in the failure to take up child allowances, which further drives the household into poverty (De Schutter, 2022b).

At a policy level, leaving no child behind will mean proofing and monitoring policies to ensure that they are designed and delivered in ways which reach the most disadvantaged children. Access to ECEC for children from disadvantaged backgrounds could be prioritised where supply is scarce. Additional resources could be allocated to ECEC facilities and schools in disadvantaged areas, and the provision of leisure facilities for such areas could be increased. Special outreach health programmes to disadvantaged communities and families could be designed. Barriers such as costs could be addressed by subsidising facilities or providing them free-of-charge for children from low-income households. Thus, depending on the issue, sometimes it will be best to develop a neighbourhood or local/regional approach targeting the most disadvantaged communities, and in other instances an approach targeting low-income households will be more appropriate. In general, the two approaches will operate most effectively in combination.[3] When implementing a strategy that focuses on children experiencing the severest disadvantage, it is important to ensure that this does not become a substitute for investing in prevention measures and in policies aimed at ensuring that vulnerability does not worsen. Such a strategy should also ensure that these children have access to the same universal services as all other children. Indeed, some services need to be provided to all/most children where this is the only way to avoid stigmatisation (Frazer et al, 2020). A major political advantage of focusing on ensuring access of children from disadvantaged backgrounds to universal provision is that middle-class taxpayers whose own children attend this provision will have a vested interest in ensuring that this provision is of a high quality and will thus be more inclined to support it.

Putting children's rights at the heart of strategies to end IGPP

Living in poverty undermines people's human rights. Grounding the fight against poverty in human rights, and particularly in

---

[3] An example of such a dual approach can be seen in relation to education in Ireland, where the additional costs of education are addressed through the Back to School Clothing and Footwear Allowance which is aimed at low-income households with children, while at the same time there is also a neighbourhood approach targeting schools in disadvantaged areas, the Delivering Opportunities in Schools programme.

the UN Convention on the Rights of the Child, fundamentally changes its nature and promotes a comprehensive approach to combating child poverty. It requires that we see poverty reduction not as charity but as a legal obligation imposed on governments, who should be held accountable for results. The relationship between people in poverty and public service providers is transformed: it is re-described as a relationship between rights holders and duty bearers, thus promoting empowerment and ensuring that beneficiaries have access to independent recourse mechanisms, including the courts, to file claims against instances of exclusion. This in turn provides a safeguard, however imperfect, against corruption and discrimination; and, by reducing the stigma attached to the claiming of benefits, it may significantly reduce the rates of non-take-up (De Schutter, 2022b). Finally, a human rights-based approach to poverty reduction includes a requirement of participation of people in poverty in the design, implementation and evaluation of the policies that affect them: this should ensure that the policies will be better informed by the lived experience of people in poverty, thus improving their effectiveness (Eurochild and EAPN, 2013).

Strikingly, children's rights have been at the heart of major approaches by the EU to combating child poverty and promoting child well-being. The 2013 EU Recommendation makes it a core principle to

> address child poverty and social exclusion from a children's rights approach, in particular by referring to the relevant provisions of the Treaty on the European Union, the Charter of Fundamental Rights of the European Union and the UN Convention on the Rights of the Child, making sure that these rights are respected, protected and fulfilled. (European Commission, 2013)

The Recommendation establishing the European Child Guarantee uses a similar wording (Council of the EU, 2021).

The importance and many advantages of adopting a children's rights approach is repeatedly stressed by a broad range of organisations working with children, such as Eurochild and the EU Alliance for Investing in Children (Eurochild, 2022; EU Alliance for Investing in Children, 2020a).

Improving research and data collection, promoting child mainstreaming, enhancing monitoring and reporting and setting targets

The design of effective anti-poverty strategies requires that we improve our understanding of IGPP, especially in the developing world, where the research gaps are the most significant. Research must continue to take a multidimensional approach, and study less researched areas such as mental health and neighbourhood effects. There is a need to emphasise non-material transfers in developing countries and to explore more closely the mechanisms by which poverty is perpetuated from one generation to the next. Data are essential to ensure better mapping of child poverty and IGPP, to enhance evidence-based policy development and to ensure effective monitoring and reporting on progress. In relation to children this should be informed by a child-mainstreaming approach which considers how every policy affects children. As Atkinson and Marlier have pointed out: 'This approach should be not simply to disaggregate by age but to ask "what indicators would best serve the needs of children?". There is, for example, a good case to be made for considering measures of child health, child development or, more broadly "child well-being".' They have also stressed that 'in considering child-focused indicators, it is important to recognise that there may be differences between the interests of children and the interests of the parents who often make choices on their behalf' (Atkinson and Marlier, 2010; see also Marlier et al, 2007).

One of the recurrent problems with efforts to combat poverty is the practical implementation of policies. Too often there is a gap between what is intended and what actually happens. Effective monitoring and accountability systems may ensure that the policies implemented to combat IGPP and child poverty are regularly monitored and improved so as to ensure that they are efficiently and effectively delivered, that they are adequate and that access to them is ensured for children in vulnerable situations (Frazer et al, 2020). The more rigorously monitoring is undertaken and the more visibly it is reported, the greater the pressure on political systems to maintain a priority and ensure effective delivery.

Setting targets for the reduction of poverty can be an important element both in increasing the visibility and political importance of efforts and in enhancing monitoring and reporting. In 2010, as part of the Europe 2020 strategy for smart, sustainable and inclusive growth, the EU set a specific and time-bound target for the EU as a whole, to be achieved by 2020: lifting at least 20 million people out of the risk of poverty and social exclusion in the EU (European Council, 2010). This target was measured on the basis of the 'at-risk-of-poverty-or-social-exclusion' indicator, according to which people are at risk of poverty or social exclusion if they live in a household that is at risk of poverty and/or severely materially deprived and/or (quasi-)jobless (see Frazer et al, 2014 for a discussion of this indicator; and European Commission, 2019 for a thorough analysis of progress EU Member States made towards the 2020 target between 2010 and 2019). In 2021, the EU agreed a new target to be achieved by 2030: to reduce the number of people at risk of poverty or social exclusion by at least 15 million, of which at least 5 million should be children (European Commission, 2021a).[4] By October 2022, 19 Member States had decided, on a voluntary basis, to set national targets for the reduction

---

[4]   The at-risk-of-poverty-or-social-exclusion indicator used for the 2030 target is also an aggregate measure which combines poverty risk, severe deprivation and (quasi-)joblessness. However, compared with the indicator used for the 2020 target, the definitions of the deprivation and (quasi-)joblessness measures have been changed. For the exact definition, see Social Protection Committee (2022a).

of child poverty or social exclusion (for a presentation of these targets, see Social Protection Committee, 2022b).

Ensuring adequate participation

Ensuring the participation of people experiencing poverty in the design of poverty-reduction strategies is key both to their legitimacy and to their effectiveness. As noted by the CESCR,

> a policy or programme that is formulated without the active and informed participation of those affected is most unlikely to be effective. Although free and fair elections are a crucial component of the right to participate, they are not enough to ensure that those living in poverty enjoy the right to participate in key decisions affecting their lives. (UN Committee on Economic, Social and Cultural Rights, 2001, para 12)

The Guiding Principles on extreme poverty and human rights provide that

> States must ensure the active, free, informed and meaningful participation of persons living in poverty at all stages of the design, implementation, monitoring and evaluation of decisions and policies affecting them. This requires capacity-building and human rights education for persons living in poverty, and the establishment of specific mechanisms and institutional arrangements, at various levels of decision-making, to overcome the obstacles that such persons face in terms of effective participation. Particular care should be taken to fully include the poorest and most socially excluded persons. (OHCHR, 2012, para 38)

The Guiding Principles also call on countries to 'adopt and implement a comprehensive national strategy and plan of action to eliminate poverty, framed in human rights terms'. These strategies and plans 'should be devised and periodically reviewed through a transparent, inclusive, participatory and gender-sensitive process'. The process by which they are devised, and their content, 'should pay particular attention to vulnerable or marginalised groups. States should define and publicise opportunities for participation and information about proposed policy measures should be disseminated widely and in an accessible manner' (OHCHR, 2012, para 104).

Low levels of education, lack of self-confidence, poor access to information, the difficulty to organise collectively, time poverty and lack of trust in the officials or institutions organising the consultation are all important obstacles that people in poverty face in exercising their right to take part in the conduct of public affairs. Yet, ensuring such effective participation is the only way to break the vicious cycle in which people in poverty are trapped: as long as they will remain underrepresented in decision making, the policies that are ostensibly meant to support them will be poorly informed about the reality of the challenges they face and, in particular, may not reach the most marginalised groups (Lansdown, 2011). In contrast, adequate participation, informed by the specific obstacles to participation that people in poverty may face, can significantly improve the effectiveness of the delivery of public services. An experiment to promote community-based monitoring of public primary healthcare providers in Uganda, for instance, illustrated how improved participation led to large increases in utilisation and improved health outcomes, including reduced child mortality and increased child weight (Björkman and Svensson, 2009). The Irish Government's National Strategy on Children and Young People's Participation in Decision-Making 2015–2020 provides another example (Department of Children and Youth Affairs, 2015).

The role of participation in improving our understanding of poverty is perhaps best illustrated by the 'Hidden Dimensions of Poverty' research project, co-led by ATD Fourth World and Oxford University between 2017 and 2019. The research involved 1,091 participants across six countries (including 665 adults and children in poverty), both from rich countries (France, the UK and the US) and from the global South (Bangladesh, Bolivia and Tanzania) (Bray et al, 2019). The report was based on the 'Merging of Knowledge' methodology, defined as a process in which academics, practitioners (activists, social workers) and people in poverty first build knowledge independently in peer meetings and then merge these various sources of knowledge (respectively from science, from practice and from the lived experience of poverty) in order to develop new insights into poverty: the process recognises and values the specific understandings gained for the experience of poverty, and exposes each participant to the knowledge and experience of others 'in order to build knowledge that is more complete and greater than the sum of its parts'.[5]

The process led to the identification of six 'hidden dimensions' of poverty. These dimensions are called 'hidden' because they go beyond lack of decent work, insufficient and insecure income, and material and social deprivation, which are the more classic forms of deprivation referred to both in the money–metric and in the multidimensional approaches to poverty.

These hidden dimensions of poverty fall into two groups. They relate, first, to what the research describes as the *core experience of poverty*, conceptualised as a mix of anguish and agency: they are referred to as 'suffering in body, mind and heart' ('experiencing intense physical, mental and emotional suffering accompanied by a sense of powerlessness to do anything about it'); 'disempowerment' (defined as 'lack of control and dependency on others resulting from severely

---

[5]   See the 'Guidelines for the Merging of Knowledge and Practices when working with people living in situations of poverty and social exclusion', available at: www.atd-fourthworld.org/wp-content/uploads/sites/5/2021/10/2021-09-08-ATDFourthWorld-GuidelinesMergingKnowledge.pdf

constrained choices'); and 'struggle and resistance' (the 'ongoing struggle to survive, which includes resisting and counteracting the effects of the many forms of suffering brought on by privations, abuse, and lack of recognition'). The second group of 'hidden dimensions of poverty' is *relational*: they are referred to as social maltreatment ('people in poverty are negatively perceived and treated badly by other individuals and informal groups', 'behaviour towards people in poverty is characterised by prejudicial negative judgements, stigma and blame'), institutional maltreatment ('the failure of national and international institutions, through their actions or inaction, to respond appropriately and respectfully to the needs and circumstances of people in poverty, and thereby ... ignor[ing], humiliat[ing] and harm[ing] them') and unrecognised contributions ('The knowledge and skills of people living in poverty are rarely seen, acknowledged or valued. Often, individually and collectively, people experiencing poverty are wrongly presumed to be incompetent'). These dimensions are described as 'relational' because they result from how people who are not living in poverty affect the lives of people in poverty, either by ignorance or by prejudice. This links these hidden dimensions of poverty with a definition of poverty based on 'social exclusion': the idea underlying both is that poverty does not have its source in the failings of the person living in poverty but, rather, in the inadequate design of institutions or policies that, for instance, continue to tolerate IGPP, to ignore qualifications acquired by practice rather than formally recognised in diplomas or to undervalue the innovations from people in poverty, particularly the solidarity mechanisms they establish to cope with deprivation.

The 'Hidden Dimensions of Poverty' research illustrates how participation is important not only for the design and implementation of poverty-reduction strategies but also to guide the methodological choices concerning data collection and poverty measurement. Indeed, as noted by the UN Special Rapporteur on the right to adequate housing, those concerned (such as, among the most marginalised groups, the homeless) 'are best placed to ensure that methods of measurement are accurate and inclusive and at the same time sensitive to their circumstances' (Farha, 2015, para 73). This was also a recommendation of Tony Atkinson, addressed to the World Bank, expressing a robust scepticism towards measurements of poverty that would be exclusively money-centric and relying on criteria distinct from the lived experiences of people in poverty. He urged the Bank to 'explore the use of subjective assessments of personal poverty status (in "quick" surveys of poverty), and of the minimum consumption considered necessary to avoid extreme poverty, as an aid to interpreting the conclusions drawn from the global poverty estimates'; and he insisted that such an 'extended listening exercise ... should make sure that the voices heard include those of children' (Atkinson, 2017, p 138). In order to ensure that such participation is effective, human rights mechanisms, including national human rights institutions, should cooperate with national statistical offices to ensure that the methodologies adopted in a country to measure poverty are adequately informed by the experiences of the poor.[6]

The EU also recognises the importance of promoting the participation of children and their parents in decision making that affects their lives as a key element in developing

---

[6] A note by the OHCHR recommends 'facilitating participation of the population, especially disadvantaged and marginalised members of society and other relevant stakeholders in the measurement process. Participation is a fundamental principle of human rights. There are already a number of collaborative efforts involving national statistical offices, representatives of population groups and national human rights institutions, such as ... in the Philippines on indigenous peoples, and in Bolivia on economic and social rights. This would require a more institutionalised partnership between official statistics and the human rights community, such as through participation of National Human Rights Institutions (NHRIs) or civil society organisations' (United Nations Economic and Social Council, 2015, para.7(c)).

more effective responses to poverty and social exclusion. It is a feature of the 2013 EU Recommendation on Investing in Children (European Commission, 2013), of the EU Recommendation on the European Child Guarantee (Council of the EU, 2021) and of the EU Strategy on the Rights of the Child (European Commission, 2021c). It is also strongly emphasised by organisations working with families and children. Eurochild and EAPN emphasise the right of children to be heard, and argue that just as children's participation is crucial, so too is involving their parents. Only by talking to parents living in poverty can the real obstacles and challenges on how to improve living conditions be understood, service deliverers be held to account and more effective solutions be developed. Parents should be involved directly in the decisions that are made over their lives and in developing their own solutions – through personalised, tailored support approaches and integrated services, but also as a collective in shaping the principal policy solutions (Eurochild and EAPN, 2013; see also ATD Fourth World, 2020; COFACE, 2020b).

Ensuring effective participation of people in poverty in the design and implementation of the policies that affect them requires taking into account the specific hurdles they face (Frazer et al, 2020; Guio et al, 2021). To overcome barriers to participation, professionals could be trained to adopt a community-development approach and see children, parents and local community organisations as partners rather than merely as beneficiaries of services designed without them. Sufficient time and space should be made for participation, and trust should be built over time. The language used should be accessible. Community members could be specially appointed to facilitate participation, and trained to that effect. And participation should be incentivised by providing assurances to participants that their voices matter – in other terms, that the concerns they express or suggestions they make will be taken into account.

Foster stronger links between poverty and environment agendas

Combating IGPP is inextricably tied in with combating climate change and promoting environmental sustainability: people in poverty are the most directly affected by the failure of governments to take bolder action to address environmental breakdown, and the reduction of inequalities is an essential component of such action, if it is to be legitimate and well informed by the experience of people in poverty (see Chapter Two, in section 'Environmental shocks' and Chapter Three, in section 'Efforts to achieve an environmentally sustainable future undermined'). Environmental sustainability must therefore become a central objective of eradicating poverty. Furthermore, reining in excessive resource consumption by the wealthiest 10% of the world's population would allow the poorest to emerge from poverty and help that ensure we remain within planetary boundaries (Paul, 2021). Thus, making progress on the one is crucial to making progress on the other. Given that these are the two most fundamental challenges facing the future of the world, it is essential that all those working and campaigning on these two issues combine their efforts to work together for the changes needed to build a fairer, more sustainable and poverty-free future. Equally important is that policy makers ensure that the development and implementation of their anti-poverty and environmental sustainability policies are closely linked and mutually reinforcing.

Conclusion

The escape from poverty must have children and their families at its heart. Because poverty disproportionately affects households with children, children are twice as likely to live in extreme poverty as adults. Globally, approximately 800 million children aged 0–18 years are subsisting below a poverty line of US$3.20 a day, and one billion children are experiencing multidimensional poverty, with multiple deprivations in the areas of health, nutrition, education or standards of living, including housing (ILO and UNICEF, 2023). This is not because parents are not caring for them. It is a failure not of families, but of governments: 1.77 billion children aged 0–18 years lack access to a child or family cash benefit, a fundamental pillar of a social protection system (ILO and UNICEF, 2023).

The failure to invest more in children by providing more support and better access to essential services to households facing poverty imposes huge costs on society: calculations taking into account the productivity returns of a more skilled and healthy workforce (which would be expected to grow over time), as practised in the 'Marginal Value of Public Funds' approach (Hendren and Sprung-Keyser, 2020), or other such methods of assessing public investment, show the long-term losses to be considerable.

In spite of this, the political powerlessness of people in poverty and a failure to listen to their voices and experiences as well as the short time horizon characteristic of political decision making are still delaying action in this regard. An equally powerful factor obstructing change is the fallacious tendency to blame poverty on dysfunctional families or, even worse, on a culture within certain sub-groups of society which is opposed to work (a thesis sometimes expressed with racist overtones). This means that the children of today's children growing up in poverty will also grow up in poverty. In this book we have debunked the myths and excuses impeding action and we have argued instead that a range of mechanisms operate to perpetuate poverty from one generation to the next. Vicious cycles operate, diminishing life chances for children raised in poverty. Yet, there is no excuse for the perpetuation of these vicious cycles: we know the range of policies and actions that are needed to break them.

The ideal of equal opportunities is a myth in a society in which stark income and wealth differences persist: as Tony Atkinson was fond of saying, if you want equality of opportunities, you must first achieve equality of outcomes. Breaking the vicious cycles requires that the fight against child poverty and IGPP is defined as a top political priority. Given the damage that poverty does to people's lives, to social cohesion, to the economy and to environmental sustainability, we can imagine no objective more urgent or worthwhile pursuing.

References

Abramo, L., Cecchini, S. and Morales, B. (2019), *Social Programmes, Poverty Eradication and Labour Inclusion. Lessons from Latin America and the Caribbean*, CEPAL (LC/PUB.2019/5-P).

Acquah, D. and Thévenon, O. (2020), 'Delivering evidence based services for all vulnerable families – a review of main policy issues', *Social, Employment and Migration Working Papers*, 243, OECD, Paris. www.oecd-ilibrary.org/social-issues-migration-health/delivering-evidence-based-services-for-all-vulnerable-families_1bb808f2-en

Adrian, N., Barnett, B., Bunn, L., Galecki, M., Ginn, J. and Plumley, B. (2020), *Climate Change and Child Poverty in OECD Countries*, The Robert M. La Follette School of Public Affairs, University of Wisconsin, Madison. https://lafollette.wisc.edu/outreach-pub lic-service/

Afrobarometer (2017), Highlights of round 6 survey findings from 36 African countries. www.afrobarometer.org

Aigner, D.J. and Cain, G.G. (1977), 'Statistical theories of discrimination in labor markets', *Industrial and Labor Relations Review*, 30(2), pp 175–187.

Akter, S. and Mallick, B. (2013), 'The poverty–vulnerability–resilience nexus: evidence from Bangladesh', *Ecological Economics*, 96, pp 114–124. https://doi.org/10.1016/j.ecolecon.2013.10.008

Alesina, A. and Glaeser, E.L. (2004), *Fighting Poverty in the US and Europe: A World of Difference*, Oxford University Press, Oxford.

Alesina, A. and La Ferrara, E. (2000), 'Participation in heterogeneous communities', *Quarterly Journal of Economics*, 115(3), pp 847–904.

Alesina, A., Hohmann, S., Michalopoulos, S. and Papaioannou, E. (2019), 'Intergenerational mobility in Africa', *National Bureau of Economic Research Working Paper*, 25534. www.nber.org/papers/w25534

Allen, M.R., Dube, O.P., Solecki, W., Aragón-Durand, F., Cramer ,W., Humphreys, S., Kainuma, M., Kala, J., Mahowald, N., Mulugetta, Y., Perez, R., Wairiu, M. and Zickfeld K. (2018), 'Framing and context', in V. Masson-Delmotte, P. Zhai, H.-O. Pörtner, D. Roberts, J. Skea, P.R. Shukla, A. Pirani, W. Moufouma-Okia, C. Péan, R. Pidcock, S. Connors, J.B.R. Matthews, Y. Chen, X. Zhou, M.I. Gomis, E. Lonnoy, T. Maycock, M. Tignor and T. Waterfield (eds), *Global Warming of 1.5°C. An IPCC Special Report on the impacts of global warming of 1.5°C above pre-industrial levels and related global greenhouse gas emission pathways, in the context of strengthening the global response to the threat of climate change, sustainable development, and efforts to eradicate poverty*, Cambridge University Press, Cambridge, UK and New York, pp 49–92. https://doi.org/10.1017/9781009157940.003

Allport, G.W. (1954), *The Nature of Prejudice*, Addison-Wesley, Cambridge, MA.

Alon, S. and Malamud, O. (2014), 'The impact of Israel's class-based affirmative action policy on admission and academic outcomes', *Economic of Education Review*, 40, pp 123–139.

Alston, P. (2015), *Report of the Special Rapporteur on Extreme Poverty and Human Rights to the Twenty-ninth Session of the Human Rights Council*, UN doc. A/HRC/29/31 (26 May 2015), United Nations, New York.

Alston, P. (2020), *The Parlous State of Poverty Eradication. Report of the Special Rapporteur on Extreme Poverty and Human Rights to the Forty-fourth Session of the Human Rights Council*, UN doc. A/HRC/44/40, United Nations, New York.

Amoly, E., Dadvand, P., Forns, J., López-Vicente, M., Basagaña, X., Julvez, J., Alvarez-Pedrerol, M., Nieuwenhuijsen, M.J. and Sunyer, J. (2014), 'Green and blue spaces and behavioral development in Barcelona schoolchildren: the BREATHE project', *Environmental Health Perspectives*, 122(12), pp 1–34.

Appadurai, A. (2004), 'The capacity to aspire: culture and the terms of recognition', in V. Rao and M. Walton (eds), *Culture and Public Action*, Stanford University Press, Paolo Alto, CA, pp 59–84. https://gsdrc.org/document-library/the-capacity-to-aspire-culture-and-the-terms-of-recognition/

Araujo, M.C., Bosch, M. and Schady, N. (2017), 'Can cash transfers help households escape an inter-generational poverty trap?' *National Bureau for Economic Research Working Paper*, 22670, Washington, DC.

ARC-CRSA (Alternate Report Coalition – Children's Rights South Africa) (2016), *Alternate Report Coalition – Children's Rights South Africa*. https://tbinternet.ohchr.org/Treaties/CRC/Shared%20Documents/ZAF/INT_CRC_NGO_ZAF_24898_E.pdf

Arrow, K.J. (1973), 'The theory of discrimination', *Discrimination in Labor Markets*, 3(10), pp 3–33.

Asfaw, S., Pickmans, R., Alfani, F. and Davis, B.N. (2016), *Productive Impact of Ethiopia's Social Cash Transfer Pilot Programme A from Protection to Production (PtoP) report*, Food and Agriculture Organization (FAO), Rome.

Asher, S., Novosad, P. and Rafkin, C. (2021), *Intergenerational Mobility in India: New Methods and Estimates across Time, Space, and Communities*. https://paulnovosad.com/pdf/anr-india-mobility.pdf

Asian Development Bank (2012), *Special Evaluation Study: ADB Social Protection Strategy 2001*.

ATD Fourth World (2004), *How Poverty Separates Parents and Children: A Challenge to Human Rights – A Study by ATD Fourth World*, Fourth World Publications, Méry-sur-Oise. www.revue-quartmonde.org/9973?file=1

ATD Fourth World (2016), 'France bans discrimination on the grounds of social conditions' (2 August).

ATD Fourth World (2020), *Submission to the European Commission's Consultation on the Child Guarantee Initiative*, European Commission, Brussels. https://ec.europa.eu/info/law/better-regulation/have-your-say/initiatives/12565-European-Child-Guarantee-/F584018

ATD Quart Monde and Changement pour l'Egalité (2017), *Nos ambitions pour l'école*, ATD Quart Monde & Changement pour l'Egalité, Brussels. https://atd-quartmonde.be/cms/wp-content/uploads/2018/03/NosAmbitionsPourEcole-BrochureWeb.pdf

Atkinson, A.B. (2015), *Inequality: What Can Be Done?* Harvard University Press, Cambridge, MA and London.

Atkinson, A.B. (2017), *Monitoring Global Poverty. Report of the Commission on Global Poverty*, The World Bank, Washington DC. https://openknowledge.worldbank.org/bitstream/handle/10986/25141/9781464809613.pdf

Atkinson, A.B. and Marlier, E. (2010), *Analysing and Measuring Social Inclusion in a Global Context*, United Nations Department of Economic and Social Affairs, New York. www.un.org/esa/soc dev/publications/measuring-social-inclusion.pdf

Attanasio, O. and Gómez, L. (eds) (2004), *Evaluación del impacto del programa Familias en Acción: subsidios condicionados a la red de apoyo social. Informe del primer seguimiento (ajustado)*, National Planning Department, Bogotá, March. http://discovery.ucl.ac.uk/14764/1/14764.pdf

Attanasio, O., Fitzsimons, E., Gomez, A., Gutiérrez, M.I., Meghir, C. and Mesnard, A. (2010), 'Children's schooling and work in the presence of a conditional cash transfer program in rural Colombia', *Economic Development and Cultural Change*, 58(2), pp 181–210.

Babones, S.J. (2008), 'Income inequality and population health: correlation and causality', *Social Science & Medicine*, 66(7), pp 1614–1626.

Balestra, C. and Tonkin, R. (2018), 'Inequalities in household wealth across OECD countries: evidence from the OECD Wealth Distribution Database', *OECD Statistics Working Paper*, 2018/01, OECD Publishing, Paris. https://doi.org/10.1787/7e1bf673-en

Banerjee, A., Hanna, R., Kreindler, G.E. and Olken, B.A. (2017), 'Debunking the stereotype of the lazy welfare recipient: evidence from cash transfer programs worldwide', *The World Bank Research Observer*, 32(2), Oxford University Press, Oxford.

Baptista, I., Guio, A., Marlier, E. and Perista, P. (2023), *Access for children in need to the key services covered by the European Child Guarantee: An analysis of policies in the 27 EU Member States*. European Social Policy Analysis Network (ESPAN), Publications Office of the European Union, Luxembourg.

Barboza Solís, C., Kelly-Irving, M., Fantin, R., Darnaudéry, M., Torrisani, J., Lang, T. and Delpierre, C. (2015), 'Adverse childhood experiences and physiological wear-and-tear in midlife: findings from the 1958 British birth cohort', *Proceedings of the National Academy of Sciences of the United States of America*, 112(7), pp E738–E746.

Bárcena Martín, E., Blázquez Cuesta, M., Budría, S. and Moro Egido, A.I. (2017), 'Child deprivation and social benefits: Europe in cross-national perspective'. *Socio-Economic Review*, 15(4), pp 717–744.

Bartlett, S. (1998), 'Does inadequate housing perpetuate children's poverty?' *Childhood*, 5(4), pp 403–420. www.researchgate.net/publication/240697311_Does_Inadequate_Housing_Perpetuate_Children%27s_Poverty

Basant, R. and Sen, G. (2020), 'Quota-based affirmative action in higher education: impact on other backward classes in India', *The Journal of Development Studies*, 56(1), pp 1–25.

Bastagli, F., Hagen-Zanker, J., Harman, L., Barca, V., Sturge, G. and Schmidt, T., with Pellerano, L. (2016), *Cash Transfers: What Does the Evidence Say? A Rigorous Review of Programme Impact and of the Role of Design and Implementation Features*, Overseas Development Institute (ODI), London.

Becker, G. (1964), *Human Capital: A Theoretical and Empirical Analysis, with Special Reference to Education*, University of Chicago Press, Chicago.

Becker, G. and Tomes, N. (1986), 'Human capital and the rise and fall of families', *Journal of Labor Economics*, 4, pp S1–S39.

Bellani, L. and Bia, M. (2017), 'The impact of growing up poor in Europe', in A.B. Atkinson, A.-C. Guio and E. Marlier (eds), *Monitoring Social Inclusion in Europe*, Eurostat, Luxembourg, pp 449–462. https://liser.elsevierpure.com/en/publications/the-impact-of-growing-up-poor-in-europe

Berg, A. and Ostry, J.D. (2011), 'Inequality and unsustainable growth: two sides of the same coin?', *IMF Staff Discussion Note* 11/08, International Monetary Fund, Washington, DC.

Berhane G., Gilligan D.O., Hoddinott J., Kumar N. and Taffesse A.S. (2014), 'Can social protection work in Africa? The Impact of Ethiopia's productive safety net programme', *Economic Development and Cultural Change*, 63(1), pp 1–26. https://doi.org/10.1086/677753

Bernard, T., Dercon, S., Orkin, K. and Seyoum Taffesse, A. (2014), *The Future in Mind: Aspirations and Forward-Looking Behaviour in Rural Ethiopia*, Centre for the Study of African Economies, University of Oxford, Oxford. www.csae.ox.ac.uk/papers/the-future-in-mind-aspirations-and-forward-looking-behaviour-in-rural-ethiopia

Bertrand, M. and Whitmore Schanzenback, D. (2009), 'Time use and food consumption', *American Economic Review: Papers & Proceedings*, 99(2), pp 170–176.

Bharadwaj, N.D. (2016), 'The relationship between poverty and the environment', *Voices of Youth*, 5 November. www.voicesofyouth.org/blog/relationship-between-poverty-and-environment

Biggs, B., King, L., Basu, S. and Stuckler, D. (2010), 'Is wealthier always healthier? The impact of national income level, inequality, and poverty on public health in Latin America', *Social Science & Medicine*, 71(2), pp 266–273. https://pubmed.ncbi.nlm.nih.gov/20471147/

Bird, K. and Higgins, K. (2011), 'Stopping the intergenerational transmission of poverty: research highlights and policy recommendations', *Working Paper*, 2014, Chronic Poverty Research Centre, Manchester. www.files.ethz.ch/isn/134296/WP214%20Bird%20and%20Higgins.pdf

Bird, K., Higgins, K. and McKay, A. (2010), 'Conflict, education and the intergenerational transmission of poverty in Northern Uganda', *Journal of International Development*, 22(8), pp 1183–1196. https://doi.org/10.1002/jid.1754

Björkman, M. and Svensson, J. (2009), 'Power to the people: evidence from a randomized field experiment on community-based monitoring in Uganda', *The Quarterly Journal of Economics*, 124(2), pp 735–769.

Blattman, C., Fiala, N. and Martinez, S. (2014), 'Generating skilled employment in developing countries: experimental evidence from Uganda', *Quarterly Journal of Economics*, 129, pp 697–752.

Bohoslavsky, J.P. (2018), *Report of the Independent Expert on the Effects of Foreign Debt and Other Related International Financial Obligations of States on the Full Enjoyment of Human Rights, Particularly Economic, Social and Cultural Rights, Fortieth Session of the Human Rights Council*, A/HRC/40/57, Geneva.

Bold, T., Filmer, D., Martin, G., Molina, E., Rockmore, C., Stacy, B., Svensson, J. and Wane, W. (2017), 'What do teachers know and do? Does it matter? Evidence from primary schools in Africa', *Policy Research Working Paper*, 7956, World Bank, Washington, DC.

Booysen, F. and Guvuriro, S. (2021), 'Gender differences in intra-household financial decision-making: an application of coarsened exact matching', *Journal of Risk and Financial Management*, 14(469). https://doi.org/10.3390/jrfm14100469

Bossuyt, M. (2002), 'The concept and practice of affirmative action', *Final Report Submitted in Accordance with Resolution 1998/5 of the Sub-Commission for the Promotion and Protection of Human Rights*, E/CN.4/ Sub.2/2002/21 (17 June).

Bowers, M. and Yehuda, R. (2016), 'Intergenerational transmission of stress in humans', *Neuropsychopharmacology*, 41(1), pp 232–244. www.nature.com/articles/npp2015247

Bradshaw, J. and Rees, G. (2019), 'Feasibility study for a child guarantee: policy area report on nutrition', Internal document, *Feasibility Study for a Child Guarantee (FSCG)*, European Commission, Brussels.

Bray, R., de Laat, M., Godinot, X., Ugarte, A. and Walker, R. (2019), *The Hidden Dimensions of Poverty*, Fourth World Publications, Montreuil.

Bray, R., de Laat, M., Godinot, X., Ugarte, A. and Walker, R. (2020), 'Realising poverty in all its dimensions: a six-country participatory study', *World Development*, 134(C). https://www.sciencedirect.com/science/article/abs/pii/S0305750X20301510?via%3Dihub

Buchmann, N., Field, E., Glennerster, R., Nazneen, S., Pimkina, S. and Sen, I. (2018), *Power vs Money: Alternative Approaches to Reducing Child Marriage in Bangladesh, a Randomized Control Trial*, Abdul Latif Jameel Poverty Action Lab (J-PAL). www.povertyactionlab.org/evaluation/empowering-girls-rural-bangladesh

Bueno, N. (2022), 'From productive work to capability-enhancing work: implications for labour law and policy', *Journal of Human Development and Capabilities*, 23(3), pp 354–372.

Cabane, C. and Clark, A.E. (2015), 'Childhood sporting activities and adult labour-market outcomes', *Annals of Economics and Statistics*, 119/120, Special issue on health and labour economics (December 2015), pp 123–148. www.jstor.org/stable/10.15609/annaeconstat2009.119-120.123

Cadinu, M., Maass, A., Rosabianca, A. and Kiesner, J. (2005), 'Why do women underperform under stereotype threat?', *Psychological Science*, 16(7), pp 572–578.

Camilo de Oliveira, A., Andrade, M.V., Resende, A.C.C., Ribas, R., Rodrigues, C. and Rodrigues, L. (2007), 'Primeiros resultados da análise da linha de base da pesquisa de avaliação de impacto do programa Bolsa Família', in J. Vaitsman and R. Paes-Sousa (eds), *Avaliação de políticas e programas do MDS: resultados*, vol. 2, Ministry of Social Development and Hunger Alleviation, Brasilia, pp 19–68.

Canvin, K., Jones, C., Marttila, A., Burström, B. and Whitehead, M. (2007), 'Can I risk using public services? Perceived consequences of seeking help and health care among households living in poverty: qualitative study', *Journal of Epidemiology and Community Health*, 61, 984–989. doi: 10.1136/jech.2006.058404

Capuano, A. (2017), 'The meaning of "social origin" in international human rights treaties: a critique of the CESCR's approach to "social origin" discrimination in the ICESCR and its (ir)relevance to national contexts such as Australia', *New Zealand Journal of Employment Relations*, 41, pp 91–112.

Carneiro, P., Løken, K.V. and Salvanes, K.G. (2015), 'A flying start? Maternity leave benefits and long-run outcomes of children', *Journal of Political Economy*, 123(2), pp 365–412.

Case, A. and Deaton, A. (2020), *Deaths of Despair and the Future of Capitalism*, Princeton: Princeton University Press.

Cassio, L., with Blasko, Z. and Szczepanikova, A. (2021), *Poverty and Mindsets: How Poverty and Exclusion over Generations Affect Aspirations, Hope and Decisions, and how to Address It*, Publications Office of the European Union, Luxembourg. https://publicati ons.jrc.ec.europa.eu/repository/handle/JRC124759

Chai, Y., Nandi, A. and Heymann, J. (2018), 'Does extending the duration of legislated paid maternity leave improve breastfeeding practices? Evidence from 38 low-income and middle-income countries', *BMJ Global Health*, 3(5), e001032. https://doi.org/ 10.1136/bmjgh-2018-001032

Chaitkin, S., Cantwell, N., Gale, C., Milligan, I., Flagothier, C., O'Kane, C. and Connelly, G. (2017), *Towards the Right Care for Children. Orientations for Reforming Alternative Care Systems. Africa, Asia, Latin America* (European Commission and SOS Children's Villages International).

Chetty, R., Hendren, N. and Katz, L. (2016), 'The effects of exposure to better neighborhoods on children: new evidence from the Moving to Opportunity Project', *American Economic Review*, 106(4), pp 855–902.

Chetty, R., Hendren, N., Kline, P. and Saez, E. (2014), 'Where is the land of opportunity? The geography of intergenerational mobility in the United States', *The Quarterly Journal of Economics*, 129(4), pp 1553–1623. https://academic.oup.com/qje/article/ 129/4/1553/1853754

Chetty, R., Stepner, M., Abraham, S., Lin, S., Scuderi, B., Turner, N., Bergeron, A. and Cutler, D. (2016), 'The association between income and life expectancy in the United States. 2001–2014', *Journal of the American Medical Association*, 315(16), pp 1750–1766.

Chmielewski, A.K. (2019), 'The global increase in the socioeconomic achievement gap, 1964 to 2015', *American Sociological Review*, 84(3), pp 517–544. https://doi.org/10.1177/0003122419847165

Christensen, M.-B., Hallum, C., Maitland, A., Parrinello, Q. and Putaturo, C. (2023), *Survival of the Richest – How We Must Tax the Super-rich Now to Fight Inequality*, Oxfam International, Oxford. https://oxfamilibrary.openrepository.com/bitstream/handle/10546/621477/bp-survival-of-the-richest-160123-en.pdf

Chzhen, Y. (2014), 'Child poverty and material deprivation in the European Union during the Great Recession', *Innocenti Working Paper*, 2014–06, UNICEF Office of Research, Florence, Italy.

Chzhen, Y. and Bradshaw, J. (2012), 'Lone parents, poverty and policy in the European Union', *Journal of European Social Policy*, 22(5), pp 487–506. https://doi.org/10.1177/0958928712456578

Cingano, F. (2014), 'Trends in income inequality and its impact on economic growth', *OECD Social, Employment and Migration Working Papers*, 163, OECD Publishing, Paris. http://dx.doi.org/10.1787/5jxrjncwxv6j-en

Clarke, C. and Thévenon, O. (2022), 'Starting unequal: how's life for disadvantaged children?' *OECD Papers on well-being and inequalities*, 6, OECD Publishing, Paris. www.oecd-ilibrary.org/social-issues-migration-health/starting-unequal_a0ec330c-en#page=54&zoom=100,84,121

COFACE (Confederation of Family Organisations in the EU) (2020a), *Child Compass 2030: Shaping a Healthy Society, Environment and Economy Fit for Children*, COFACE, Brussels. www.coface-eu.org/digitalisation/child-compass-2030-shaping-a-healthy-society-environment-and-economy-fit-for-children/

COFACE (2020b), *Submission to the European Commission's Consultation on the Child Guarantee Initiative*, European Commission, Brussels. https://ec.europa.eu/info/law/better-regulation/have-your-say/initiatives/12565-European-Child-Guarantee-/F583747

Cole, W. (2018), 'Poor and powerless: economic and political inequality in cross-national perspective, 1981–2011', *International Sociology*, 33(3), pp 21–22.

Commission des droits de la personne (Québec), *Comm. des droits de la personne v. Gauthier* (1993), 19 Commission of Human Rights Reports D/312.

Corak, M. (2013), 'Income inequality, equality of opportunity, and inter-generational mobility', *Journal of Economic Perspectives*, 27(3), pp 79–102.

Corak, M. and Piraino, P. (2011), 'The intergenerational transmission of employers', *Journal of Labor Economics*, 29(1), pp 37–68.

Corbacho, A., Frebes Cibils, V. and Lora, E. (eds) (2013), *More than Revenue: Taxation as a Development Tool*, Inter-American Development Bank and Palgrave Macmillan.

Coulibaly, S. (2022), 'Revenue effects of the global minimum corporate tax rate for African economies', *Tax Cooperation Policy Brief*, 26, South Centre, Geneva.

Council of Europe (2011), *Recommendation CM/REC(2011)12 of the Committee of Ministers to Member States on Children's Rights and Social Services Friendly to Children and Families*, Council of Europe, Strasbourg. https://rm.coe.int/168046ccea

Council of the EU (2021), *Council Recommendation (EU) 2021/1004 of 14 June 2021 Establishing a European Child Guarantee*, Council of the EU, Brussels. https://eur-lex.europa.eu/legal-content/EN/TXT/?uri=CELEX%3A32021H1004

Council of the EU (2023), *Council Recommendation of 30 January 2023 on Adequate Minimum Income Ensuring Active Inclusion 2023/C 41/01*, Council of the EU, Brussels. https://eur-lex.europa.eu/legal-content/EN/TXT/?uri=CELEX%3A32023H0203%2801%29

Curristan, S., Maître, B. and Russell, H. (2022), 'Intergenerational poverty in Ireland', *ESRI Research Series*, 150, ESRI, Dublin. www.esri.ie/publications/intergenerational-poverty-in-ireland

Dabla-Norris, E., Kochhar, K., Suphaphiphat, N., Ricka, F. and Tsounta, E. (2015), *Causes and Consequences of Income Inequality: A Global Perspective*, IMF Staff Discussion Note, International Monetary Fund, Washington, DC.

Daku, M., Raub, A. and Heymann, J. (2012), 'Maternal leave policies and vaccination coverage: a global analysis', *Social Science & Medicine (1982)*, 74(2), pp 120–124. https://doi.org/10.1016/j.socscimed.2011.10.013

Davis, J. and Mazumder, B. (2022), 'The decline in intergenerational mobility after 1980', *Federal Reserve Bank of Chicago Working Paper*, 2017–05, first published 2017, revised 14 January 2022.

De Schutter, O. (2010), *Report of the Special Rapporteur on the Right to Food, Olivier De Schutter, to the Thirteenth Session of the Human Rights Council, Addendum: Mission to Brazil (12–18 October 2009)* (A/HRC/13/33/Add.6).

De Schutter, O. (2015), 'Welfare state reform and social rights', *Netherlands Quarterly of Human Rights*, 33(2), pp 123–162.

De Schutter, O. (2021a), 'The persistence of poverty: how real equality can break the vicious cycles', *Report of the Special Rapporteur on Extreme Poverty and Human Rights*, A/76/177 (19 July), United Nations, New York. http://undocs.org/A/76/177

De Schutter, O. (2021b), *Report of the Special Rapporteur on Extreme Poverty and Human Rights to the Forty-seventh Session of the Human Rights Council, Addendum: Visit to the European Union* (A/HRC/47/36/Add.1).

De Schutter, O. (2022a), 'Banning discrimination on grounds of socio-economic disadvantage: an essential tool in the fight against poverty', *Report of the Special Rapporteur on Extreme Poverty and Human rights to the Seventy-seventh Session of the UN General Assembly* (A/77/157).

De Schutter, O. (2022b), 'The non-take-up of rights in the context of social protection', *Report of the Special Rapporteur on Extreme Poverty and Human rights to the Fiftieth Session of the Human Rights Council* (A/HRC/50/38).

De Schutter, O., Swinnen, J.F. and Wouters, J. (2012), 'Introduction: foreign direct investment and human development', in O. De Schutter, J. Swinnen and J. Wouters (eds), *Foreign Direct Investment and Human Development: The Law and Economics of International Investment Agreements*, Routledge, pp 1–24, London and New York.

de Vuijst, E., van Ham, M. and Kleinhans, R. (2017), 'The moderating effect of higher education on the intergenerational transmission of residing in poverty neighbourhoods', *Environment and Planning A*, 49(9), pp 2135–2154. https://doi.org/10.1177/0308518X17715638

Deininger, K. and Liu, Y. (2013), 'Welfare and poverty impacts of India's national rural employment guarantee scheme: evidence from Andhra Pradesh', *Policy Research Working Paper*, 6543, World Bank, Washington, DC.

Department of Children and Youth Affairs (2015), *National Strategy on Children and Young People's Participation in Decision-Making 2015– 2020*, Government Publications, Dublin. www.gov.ie/en/publ ication/9128db-national-strategy-on-children-and-young-peop les-participation-in-dec/

Dest, M.P. (2009), 'The impact of Brazil's Bolsa Família program on food security in Santo Antônio de Jesus, Bahia', *Independent Study Project (ISP) Collection*, 756. https://digitalcollections.sit. edu/isp_collection/756

Díaz de Sarralde, S., Carlos Garcimartín, C. and Ruiz-Huerta, J. (2010), 'The paradox of progressivity in low-tax countries: income tax in Guatemala', *CEPAL Review*, 102, pp 85–99.

Dolan, P., Peasgood, T. and White, M. (2008), 'Do we really know what makes us happy? A review of the economic literature on the factors associated with subjective well-being', *Journal of Economic Psychology*, 29(1), pp 94–122.

Dornan, P. and Woodhead, M. (2015), 'How inequalities develop through childhood: life course evidence from the Young Lives cohort study', *Innocenti Discussion Paper*, 2015–01, UNICEF Office of Research, Florence. www.unicef-irc.org/publications/ pdf/idp_2015_01(2).pdf

Doyle, J. (2010), *Misguided Kindness. Making the Right Decisions for Children in Emergencies*, Save the Children UK, London.

Drèze, J. (2019), *Sense and Solidarity: Jholawala Economics for Everyone*, online edition, Oxford Academic, Oxford. https://doi. org/10.1093/oso/9780198833468.001.0001

Duggan, A., Portilla, X.A., Filene, J.H., Shea Crowne, S., Hill, C.J., Lee, H. and Knox, V. (2018), *Implementation of Evidence-Based Early Childhood Home Visiting: Results from the Mother and Infant Home Visiting Program Evaluation*, OPRE Report # 2018–76A, Office of Planning, Research, and Evaluation, Administration for Children and Families, U.S. Department of Health and Human Services, Washington, DC.

Duncan, G.J. and Murnane, R.J. (eds) (2011), 'Introduction', *Whither Opportunity? Rising Inequality, Schools, and Children's Life Chances*, Russell Sage Foundation, New York.

Duncan, G.J. and Murnane, R.J. (2014), *Restoring Opportunity. The Crisis of Inequality and the Challenge for American Education*, Harvard Education Press & The Russell Sage Foundation, New York.

Elson, D., Balakrishnan, R. and Heintz, J. (2013), 'Public finance, maximum available resources and human rights', in A. Nolan, R. O'Connell and C. Harvey, *Human Rights and Public Finance: Budgets and the Promotion of Economic and Social Rights*, Hart Publishing, Oxford, pp 13–39.

Equinet (European Network of Equality Bodies) (2010), *Addressing Poverty and Discrimination: Two Sides of the One Coin*, Equinet Opinion. www.equineteurope.org/IMG/pdf/poverty_opinion_2010_english.pdf

Ermisch, J., Jäntti, M. and Smeeding, T.M. (eds) (2012), *From Parents to Children: the Intergenerational Transmission of Advantage*, Russell Sage Foundation, New York.

Esping-Andersen, G. (1990), *The Three Worlds of Welfare Capitalism*, Princeton University Press, Princeton.

EU Alliance for Investing in Children (2020a), *Contribution of the EU Alliance for Investing in Children to the European Commission Public Consultation on the Child Guarantee*, European Commission, Brussels. www.alliance4investinginchildren.eu/contribution-of-the-eu-alliance-for-investing-in-children-to-the-european-commission-public-consultation-on-the-child-guarantee/

EU Alliance for Investing in Children (2020b), *Joint Statement on Protecting Children and Their Families during and after the COVID19 Crisis*, EU Alliance for Investing in Children, Brussels. www.alliance4investinginchildren.eu/joint-statement-on-protectingc hildren-and-their-families-during-and-after-the-covid19-crisis/

EU Statistics on Income and Living Conditions (EU-SILC) Users' Data Base (2021).

Eurochild (2020), *Protecting Children Now and in the Future, Eurochild Public Statement on COVID-19*, Eurochild, Brussels. www.euroch ild.org/news/newsdetails/article/protecting-children-now-and-in-the-future-eurochild-public-statement-oncovid-19/?no_cache=1

Eurochild (2022), *Countering Anti-child Rights Movements in Europe: The Need for a European Mechanism*, Position paper, February 2022. https://eurochild.org/resource/position-paper-countering-anti-child-rights-movements-in-europe-the-need-for-a-european-mechanism/

Eurochild and EAPN (European Anti-Poverty Network) (2013), *Towards Children's Well-being in Europe: Explainer on Child Poverty in the EU*, Eurochild and EAPN, Brussels. www.eapn.eu/towards-children-s-well-being-in-europe-eapn-and-eurochild-s-explainer-on-child-poverty-in-the-eu-is-out-2/

European Commission (2013), *Investing in Children: Breaking the Cycle of Disadvantage*, Commission Recommendation C(2013) 778 final, European Commission, Brussels. https://eur-lex.europa.eu/legal-content/EN/TXT/PDF/?uri=CELEX:32013H0112&from=EN

European Commission (2017), *European Pillar of Social Rights*, European Commission, Brussels. https://ec.europa.eu/commission/priorities/deeper-and-fairer-economic-and-monetary-union/european-pillar-social-rights/european-pillar-social-rights-20-principles_en

European Commission (2019), *Assessment of the Europe 2020 Strategy, Joint report of the Employment Committee (EMCO) and Social Protection Committee (SPC)*, Publications Office of the European Union, Luxembourg.

European Commission (2021a), *The European Pillar of Social Rights Action Plan*, European Commission, Brussels. https://op.europa.eu/webpub/empl/european-pillar-of-social-rights/downloads/KE0921008ENN.pdf

European Commission (2021b), *Benefits of Extracurricular Activities for Children: A Focus on Social Inclusion and Children from Disadvantaged and Vulnerable Backgrounds*, Publications Office of the EU, Luxembourg. https://op.europa.eu/en/publication-detail/-/publication/c2c8d076-0a04-11ec-b5d3-01aa75ed71a1/language-en

European Commission (2021c), *EU Strategy on the Rights of the Child*, Communication from the Commission to the European Parliament, the Council, the European Economic and Social Committee and the Committee of the Regions, COM(2021) 142 final, European Commission, Brussels. https://eur-lex.eur opa.eu/legal-content/en/TXT/?uri=CELEX%3A52021DC0142

European Council (2010), *European Council 17 June 2010: Conclusions*, European Council, Brussels.

European Parliament (2016), *Report on Poverty: A Gender Perspective*, Committee on Women's Rights and Gender Equality, (2015/ 2228(INI)), European Parliament, Brussels. www.europarl.eur opa.eu/doceo/document/A-8-2016-0153_EN.pdf

Eurostat (2021), *Intergenerational Transmission of Disadvantages: Statistics*. Eurostat Statistics Explained, Data downloaded in November 2021.

Eyal, K. and Burns, J. (2016), 'Up or down? Intergenerational mental health transmission and cash transfers in South Africa', *SALDRU Working Papers* 165, Southern Africa Labour and Development Research Unit, University of Cape Town. https://econpapers. repec.org/paper/ldrwpaper/165.htm

FAO (Food and Agriculture Organization) (2017), *The Economic Case for the Expansion of Social Protection Programmes*, FAO, Rome.

FAO and WHO (World Health Organization) (2019), *Sustainable Healthy Diets. Guiding Principles*, FAO, Rome.

Farha, L. (2015), *Report of the Special Rapporteur on Adequate Housing as a Component of the Right to an Adequate Standard of Living, and on the Right to Non-discrimination in this Context*, UN doc. A/HRC/ 31/54 (30 December 2015), United Nations, New York. www. undocs.org/A/HRC/31/54

Farha, L. (2020), 'Guidelines for the implementation of the right to adequate housing', *Report of the Special Rapporteur on Adequate Housing as a Component of the Right to an Adequate Standard of Living, and on the Right to Non-discrimination in this Context*, UN doc. A/ HRC/43/43 (26 December 2019), United Nations, New York. www.undocs.org/A/HRC/43/43

Ferro, A., Kassouf, A. and Levison, D. (2010), 'The impact of conditional cash transfer programmes on household work decisions in Brazil', *Child Labor and the Transition between School and Work, Research in Labor Economics*, vol. 13, R. Akee, E. Edmonds and K. Tatsiramos (eds), Emerald Group Publishing Limited Bradford.

Frazer, H. (2020), 'COVID-19: Lessons from disadvantaged communities for EU social policy', *OSE Paper Series*, Opinion Paper 24, European Social Observatory (OSE), Brussels. www.ose.be/fr/publication/covid-19-lessons-disadvantaged-communities-eu-social-policy

Frazer, H. and Marlier, E. (2013), *Investing in Children: Breaking the Cycle of Disadvantage: A Study of National Policies*, European Social Policy Network (ESPN), European Commission, Brussels. https://op.europa.eu/en/publication-detail/-/publication/5b00fe79-b69a-4cf3-975e-4caf79bc1d06/language-en/format-PDF/source-search

Frazer, H. and Marlier, E. (2017), *Progress across Europe in the Implementation of the 2013 EU Recommendation on 'Investing in Children: Breaking the Cycle of Disadvantage: A Study of National Policies*, European Social Policy Network (ESPN), European Commission, Brussels. https://op.europa.eu/en/publication-detail/-/publication/c680a1b0-9171-11e7-b92d-01aa75ed71a1/language-en

Frazer, H., Guio, A.-C. and Marlier, E. (eds) (2020), *Feasibility Study for a Child Guarantee: Final Report*, Feasibility Study for a Child Guarantee (FSCG), Publications Office of the European Union, Luxembourg. https://op.europa.eu/en/publication-detail/-/publication/c312c468-c7e0-11ea-adf7-01aa75ed71a1/language-en

Frazer, H., Marlier, E. and Nicaise, I. (2010), 'Child poverty and social exclusion', in H. Frazer, E. Marlier and I. Nicaise (eds), *A Social Inclusion Roadmap for Europe 2020*, pp 34–94, Garant, Antwerp.

Frazer, H., Guio, A.-C., Marlier, E., Vanhercke, B. and Ward, T. (2014), 'Putting the fight against poverty and social exclusion at the heart of the EU agenda: a contribution to the Mid-Term Review of the Europe 2020 Strat,egy', *OSE Paper Series*, Research Paper 15, European Social Observatory, Brussels.

Friedman, M. (1968), 'The case for the negative income tax: a view from the right', in J.H. Bunzel (ed), *Issues of American Public Policy*, Prentice-Hall, Englewood Cliffs.

García, P.J. (2019), 'Corruption in global health: the open secret', *The Lancet*, 394(10214), pp 2119–2124.

Gassmann, F., Eszter Timár, E., van Kesteren, F., Dekkers, M. and Miroro, O. (2018), *The Business Case for Social Protection in Africa*, INCLUDE: Knowledge Platform on Inclusive Development Policies, Maastricht.

Ghislandi, S., Manachotphong, W. and Perego, V.M. (2015), 'The impact of Universal Health Coverage on health care consumption and risky behaviours: evidence from Thailand', *Health Economics, Policy, and Law*, 10(3), pp 251–266. https://doi.org/10.1017/S1744133114000334

Gibson-Davis, C., Keister, L.A. and Gennetian, L.A. (2021), 'Net worth poverty in child households by race and ethnicity, 1989–2019', *Journal of Marriage and Family*, 83(3), pp 667–682. https://doi.org/10.1111/jomf.12742

Gilens, M. (2012), *Affluence and Influence. Economic Inequality and Political Power in America*, Princeton University Press, Princeton.

Glover, D., Pallais, A. and Pariente, W. (2017), 'Discrimination as a self-fulfilling prophecy: evidence from French grocery stores', *The Quarterly Journal of Economics*, 132(3), pp 1219–1260.

Goldblatt, P., Siegrist, J., Lundberg O., Marinetti, C., Farrer, L. and Costongs, C. (eds) (2015), *Drivers for Health Equity: Improving Health Equity through Action across the Life Course. Summary of Evidence and Recommendations from the Drivers Project*, EuroHealthNet, Brussels. https://eurohealthnet.eu/sites/eurohealthnet.eu/files/publications/DRIVERS_Recommendations_rel2.pdf

González-Rozada, M. and Llerena, F. (2011), *The Effects of a Conditional Transfer Program on the Labor Market: The Human Development Bonus in Ecuador*, Inter-American Development Bank, Washington, DC. http://conference.iza.org/conference_files/worldb2011/gonzalez-rozada_m6803.pdf

Granovetter, M. (1995), *Getting a Job: A Study of Contacts and Careers*, 2nd edn, University of Chicago Press, Chicago.

Gross-Manos, D. and Bradshaw, J. (2022), 'The association between the material well-being and the subjective well-being of children in 35 countries'. *Child Indicators Research*, 15(1), pp 1–33. https://link.springer.com/article/10.1007/s12187-022-09930-8

Gugushvili, D. and Laenen, T. (2019), 'Twenty years after Korpi and Palme's "paradox of redistribution": what have we learned so far, and where should we take it from here?', *SPSW Working Paper*, 5, Centre for Sociological Research, KU Leuven, Leuven.

Guio, A.-C. (2023), 'Free school meals for all poor children in Europe: an important and affordable target?', *Children & Society*, Wiley Online Library. https://onlinelibrary.wiley.com/doi/10.1111/chso.12700

Guio, A.-C., Frazer, H. and Marlier, E. (eds) (2021), *Study on the Economic Implementing Framework of a Possible EU Child Guarantee Scheme Including Its Financial Foundation*, Second phase of the Feasibility Study for a Child Guarantee (FSCG2): Final Report, European Commission, Brussels. https://op.europa.eu/en/publication-detail/-/publication/fb5ea446-ad4e-11eb-9767-01aa75ed71a1/language-en/format-PDF/source-211627870

Guio, A.-C., Gordon, D., Marlier, E., Najera, H. and Pomati, M. (2018), 'Towards an EU measure of child deprivation', *Child Indicators Research*, 11, pp 835–860. https://doi.org/10.1007/s12187-017-9491-6

Guio, A.-C., Marlier, E., Vandenbroucke, F. and Verbunt, P. (2022), 'Differences in child deprivation across Europe: the role of in-cash and in-kind transfers', *Child Indicators Research*, 15, 2363–2388. https://doi.org/10.1007/s12187-022-09948-y

Gustafsson-Wright, E. (2013), *A Short-term Impact Evaluation of the Health Insurance Fund Program in Central Kwara State, Nigeria*, AIID and AIGHD Foundation.

Handa, S., Natali, L., Seidenfeld, D., Tembo, G. and Davis, B. (2018), 'Can unconditional cash transfers raise long-term living standards? Evidence from Zambia', *Journal of Development Economics*, 133, pp 42–65. https://doi.org/10.1016/j.jdeveco.2018.01.008

Handa, S., Park, M., Osei Darko, R., Osei-Akoto, I., Davis, B. and Daidone, S. (2014), *Livelihood Empowerment against Poverty Program Impact Evaluation*. University of North Carolina at Chapel Hill.

Hanson, J.L., Hair, N., Shen, D.G., Shi, F., Gilmore, J.H., Wolfe, B.L. and Pollak, S.D. (2013), 'Family poverty affects the rate of human infant brain growth', *PLoS One*, 8(12), e80954. https://doi.org/10.1371/journal.pone.0080954

Hanushek, E.A. and Woessmann, L. (2019), 'The economic benefits of improving educational achievement in the European Union: an update and extension', *Analytical Report*, 39, European Commission, Brussels.

Haughton, J. and Khandker, S. (2009), *Handbook on Inequality and Poverty*, World Bank, Washington, DC.

Haushofer, J. and Shapiro, J. (2016), 'The short-term impact of unconditional cash transfers to the poor: experimental evidence from Kenya', *The Quarterly Journal of Economics*, 131(4), pp 1973–2042.

Heckman, J.J. (2006), 'Skill formation and the economics of investing in disadvantaged children', *Science*, 312(5782), pp 1900–1902.

Heckman, J.J. (2007), 'The economics, technology and neuroscience of human capability formation', *Proceedings of the National Academy of Sciences*, 104, pp 13250–13255.

Heckman, J.J. (2008), 'Schools, skills, and synapses', *National Bureau of Economic Research Working Paper*, 14064, National Bureau of Economic Research, Cambridge, MA.

Heckman, J.J. and Mosso, S. (2014), 'The economics of human development and social mobility', *National Bureau of Economic Research Working Paper*, 19925, National Bureau of Economic Research, Cambridge, MA.

Heiserman, N. and Simpson, B. (2017), 'Higher inequality increases the gap in the perceived merit of the rich and poor', *Social Psychology Quarterly*, 80(3), pp 243–253.

Hendren, N. and Sprung-Keyser, B. (2020), 'A unified welfare analysis of government policies', *The Quarterly Journal of Economics*, 135(3), pp 1209–1318. https://academic.oup.com/qje/article/135/3/1209/5781614

Heymann, J., Sprague, A.R., Nandi, A., Earle, A., Batra, P., Schickedanz, A., Chung, P.J. and Raub, A. (2017), 'Paid parental leave and family wellbeing in the sustainable development era', *Public Health Reviews*, 38, 21. https://doi.org/10.1186/s40985-017-0067-2

High Level Panel of Experts on Food Security and Nutrition (HLPE) (2017), *Nutrition and food systems. A report by the High Level Panel of Experts on Food Security and Nutrition of the Committee on World Food Security*, Rome.

Hirsch, D. (2008), *Estimating the Costs of Child Poverty*, Joseph Rowntree Foundation, York. www.jrf.org.uk/report/estimating-costs-child-poverty

Hirschman, A.O. and Rothschild, M. (1973), 'The changing tolerance for income inquality in the course of economic development', *Quarterly Journal of Economics*, 87(4), pp 544–566.

Hoff, K. and Pandey, P. (2006), 'Discrimination, social identity, and durable inequalities', *American Economic Review*, 96(2), pp 206–2011.

Houses of the Oireachtas [Ireland] (2021), Equality (Miscellaneous Provisions) Bill 2021, https://data.oireachtas.ie/ie/oireachtas/bill/2021/6/eng/initiated/b0621d.pdf

Hoy, C. and Sumner, A. (2016), 'Gasoline, guns and giveaways: is there new capacity for redistribution to end three quarters of global poverty?' *CGD Working Paper 433*, Center for Global Development, Washington, DC.

Hsiao, A., Vogt, V. and Quentin, W. (2019), 'Effect of corruption on perceived difficulties in healthcare access in sub-Saharan Africa', *PLoS One*, 14(11), e0220583. https://doi.org/10.1371/journal.pone.0220583

ILO (International Labour Organization) (2020), *Global Wage Report 2020–21: Wages and Minimum Wages in the Time of COVID-19*, ILO, Geneva.

ILO and UNICEF (United Nations Children's Fund) (2021), *Child Labour: Global Estimates 2020, Trends and the Road Forward*, ILO, Geneva and UNICEF, New York. www.ilo.org/ipec/Informationresources/WCMS_797515/lang--en/index.htm

ILO and UNICEF (2023), *More than a Billion Reasons: The Urgent Need to Build Universal Social Protection for Children*, Second ILO–UNICEF Joint Report on Social Protection for Children, Geneva and New York.

Inchley, J., Currie, D., Young, T., Samdal, O., Torsheim, T., Augustson, L., Mathison, F., Aleman-Diaz, A., Molcho, M., Weber, M. and Barnekow, V. (eds) (2016), 'Growing up unequal: gender and socioeconomic differences in young people's health and well-being', *Health Behaviour in School-Aged Children (HBSC) Study (International Report from the 2013/2014 Survey)*, Health Policy for Children and Adolescents, 7, WHO, Geneva. www.euro.who.int/__data/assets/pdf_file/0003/303438/HSBC-No.7-Growing-up-unequal-Full-Report.pdf

International Monetary Fund (2014), *Fiscal Policy and Income Inequality*, Policy Paper, International Monetary Fund, Washington, DC.

Iversen, V., Krishna, A. and Sen, K. (2019), 'Beyond poverty escapes – social mobility in developing countries: a review article', *The World Bank Research Observer*, 34(2), pp 239–273. https://doi.org/10.1093/wbro/lkz003

Jackee, J.W. (2011), 'Do bilateral investment treaties promote foreign direct investment? Some hints from alternative evidence', *Virginia Journal of International Law*, 51, p 397.

Jackson, T. (2017), *Prosperity without Growth. Foundations for the Economy of Tomorrow*, Routledge, London.

Jerrim, J. and Macmillan, L. (2015), 'Income inequality, intergenerational mobility, and the Great Gatsby curve: is education the key?', *Social Forces*, 94(2), pp 505–533.

Kakwani, N.C. (1977), 'Measurement of tax progressivity: an international comparison', *The Economic Journal*, 87(345), pp 71–80.

Kaufman, W. (2011), 'A successful job search: it's all about networking', National Public Radio, 3 February. www.npr.org/2011/02/08/133474431/a-successful-job-search-its-all-about-networking

Kawachi, I. and Berkman, L.F. (eds) (2003), *Neighborhoods and Health*, Oxford University Press, New York.

Kelly, O. (2016), 'Street trees proliferate in wealthy areas, reveals city research', *The Irish Times*, Dublin. www.irishtimes.com/news/ireland/irish-news/street-trees-proliferate-in-wealthy-areas-reveals-city-research-1.2552994

Khan, Md. A., Rahaman, L. and Khan, Md. S. (2020), *Multidimensionality of Poverty: Bangladesh Perspectives*, Fourth World Publications, Pierrelaye. www.atd-fourthworld.org/wp-content/uploads/sites/5/2020/04/National-report-of-Bangladesh-Final.pdf

Korpi, W. and Palme, J. (1998), 'The paradox of redistribution and strategies of equality: welfare state institutions, inequality, and poverty in the Western countries', *American Sociological Review*, 63(5), pp 661–687.

Krishna, A. and Agarwal, S. (2017), 'Promoting social mobility in India: modes of action and types of support organizations', *Journal of South Asian Development*, 12(3), pp 236–258. https://journals.sagepub.com/doi/pdf/10.1177/0973174117733429

Krishnan, P. and Krutikova, S. (2013), 'Non-cognitive skill formation in poor neighbourhoods of urban India', *Discussion Paper*, DP9540, Center for Economic Policy Research (CEPR), London. https://papers.ssrn.com/sol3/papers.cfm?abstract_id=2291341

Kugler, A.D. and Rojas, I. (2018), 'Do CCTs improve employment and earnings in the very long-term? Evidence from Mexico', *National Bureau of Economic Research Working Paper Series*, No. 24248. DOI 10.3386/w24248. https://www.nber.org/papers/w24248

Kuznets, S. (1955), 'Economic growth and income inequality', *American Economic Review*, 45, pp 1–28.

Lancee, B. and van de Werfhorst, H. (2011), 'Income inequality and participation: a comparison of 24 European countries', *GINI discussion paper*, 6, AIAS, Amsterdam. www.uvaaias.net/uploaded_files/publications/DP6-Lancee,vdWerfhorst-2.pdf

Lansdown, G. (2011), *Every Child's Right to be Heard*, Save the Children, London. https://resourcecentre.savethechildren.net/node/5259/pdf/5259.pdf

Larson, K., Russ, S.A., Nelson, B.B., Olson, L.M. and Halfon, N. (2015), 'Cognitive ability at kindergarten entry and socioeconomic status', *Pediatrics*, 135(2), e440–8. https://pubmed.ncbi.nlm.nih.gov/25601983/

Layte, R. and Whelan, C.T. (2014), 'Who feels inferior? A test of the status anxiety hypothesis of social inequalities in health', *European Sociological Review*, 30(4), pp 525–35.

Leichenko, R. and Silva, J.A. (2014), 'Climate change and poverty: vulnerability, impacts, and alleviation strategies', *Wiley Interdisciplinary Reviews: Climate Change*, 5(4), pp 539–556. https://wires.onlinelibrary.wiley.com/doi/abs/10.1002/wcc.287

Lerch, V. and Nordenmark Severinsson, A. (2019), *Children in Alternative Care*, Feasibility Study for a Child Guarantee (FSCG), European Commission, Brussels. https://ec.europa.eu/social/main.jsp?catId=1428&langId=en

Lewer, D., Jayatunga, W., Aldridge, R.W., Edge, C., Marmot, M., Story, A. and Hayward (2020), 'Premature mortality attributable to socioeconomic inequality in England between 2003 and 2018: an observational study', *Lancet Public Health 2019*, 5(1), pp E33–E41. https://doi.org/10.1016/S2468-2667(19)30219-1

Lockwood, P. and Kunda, Z. (1997), 'Superstars and me: predicting the impact of role models on the self', *Journal of Personality and Social Psychology*, 73(1), pp 91–103.

Loury, L.D. (2006) 'Some contacts are more equal than others: informal networks, job tenure, and wages', *Journal of Labor Economics*, 24(2), pp 299–318.

Louv, R. (2009), *Last Child in the Woods: Saving our Children from Nature-Deficit Disorder*, Atlantic Books, London.

Lundberg, S.J., Pollak, R.A. and Wales, T.J. (1997), 'Do husbands and wives pool their resources? Evidence from the United Kingdom child benefit', *The Journal of Human Resources*, 32(3), pp 463–480. https://doi.org/10.2307/146179

Main, G. (2018), 'Fair shares and families: a child-focused model of intra-household sharing', *Childhood Vulnerability*, 1, pp 31–49.

Main, G. and Bradshaw, J. (2016), 'Child poverty in the UK: measures, prevalence and intra-household sharing', *Critical Social Policy*, 36(1), pp 38–61.

Maluccio, J. and Flores, R. (2005), *Impact Evaluation of a Conditional Cash Transfer Program: The Nicaraguan Red de Protección Social*, International Food Policy Research Institute (IFPRI), Washington, DC.

Maluleke, R. (2020), 'Child poverty in South Africa: a multiple overlapping deprivation analysis', UNICEF.

Mani, A., Mullainathan, S., Shafir, E. and Zhao, J. (2013), 'Poverty impedes cognitive function', *Science*, 341(6149), pp 976–980. www.science.org/doi/10.1126/science.1238041

Marinescu, I. (2018), 'No strings attached: the behavioral effects of U.S. unconditional cash transfer programs', *NBER Working Paper* 24337.

Marlier, E., Atkinson, A.B., Cantillon, B. and Nolan, B. (2007), *The EU and Social Inclusion: Facing the Challenges*, Policy Press, Bristol.

Mayer, S.E. and Lopoo, L.M. (2005), 'Has the intergenerational transmission of economic status changed?' *The Journal of Human Resources*, 40, pp 169–185.

Mazumder, B. (2005), 'The apple falls even closer to the tree than we thought: new and revised estimates of the intergenerational inheritance of earnings', in S. Bowles, H. Gintis and M.O. Groves (eds), *Unequal Chances: Family Background and Economic Success*, pp 80–99, Russell Sage Foundation, New York.

McEwen, C. and McEwen, B. (2017), 'Social structure, adversity, toxic stress, and intergenerational poverty: an early childhood model', *Annual Review of Sociology*, 43, pp 445–472. https://doi.org/10.1146/annurev-soc-060116-053252

McIsaac, E. (2018), 'Discriminating against the poor is legal. That must change', *Maytree*, 12 January.

McLaughlin, M. and Rank, M. (2018), 'Estimating the economic cost of childhood poverty in the United States', *Social Work Research*, 42(2), pp 73–83. https://academic.oup.com/swr/article/42/2/73/4956930

Michalopoulos, C., Faucetta, K., Warren, A. and Mitchell, R. (2017), *Evidence on the Long-Term Effects of Home Visiting Programs: Laying the Groundwork for Long-Term Follow-Up in the Mother and Infant Home Visiting Program Evaluation (MIHOPE)*, Office of Planning, Research and Evaluation, Washington, DC.

Miller, G.E., Chen, E. and Parker, K.J. (2011), 'Psychological stress in childhood and susceptibility to the chronic diseases of aging: moving toward a model of behavioral and biological mechanisms', *Psychological Bulletin*, 137(6), pp 959–997.

Mitchell, W.F. (1998), 'The buffer stock employment model – full employment without a NAIRU', *Journal of Economic Issues*, 32(2), pp 547–55.

Miyan, M.A. (2015), 'Droughts in Asian least developed countries: vulnerability and sustainability', *Weather and Climate Extremes*, 7, pp 8–23. www.sciencedirect.com/science/article/pii/S2212094714000632

Montero, A.L. (2016), *Investing in Children's Services Improving Outcomes*, European Social Network, Brussels. www.esn-eu.org/sites/default/files/publications/FINAL_Investing_in_Childrens_Services_WEB.pdf

Mullainathan, S. and Shafir, E. (2013), *Scarcity. The New Science of Having Less and How It Defines Our Lives*, H. Holt & Co, New York.

Munshi, K. (2011), 'Strength in numbers: networks as a solution to occupational traps', *The Review of Economic Studies*, 78(3), pp 1069–1101. https://doi.org/10.1093/restud/rdq029

Murphy, M.P. (2023), *Creating an EcoSocial Welfare Future*, Policy Press, Bristol University Press, Bristol.

Mvukiyehe, E. (2018), 'What are we learning about the impacts of public works programs on employment and violence? Early findings from ongoing evaluations in fragile states'. https://blogs.worldbank.org/impactevaluations/what-are-we-learning-about-impacts-public-works-programs-employment-and-violence-early-findings

Naher, N., Hoque, R., Hassan, M.S., Balabanova, D., Adams, A.M. and Ahmed, S.M. (2020), 'The influence of corruption and governance in the delivery of frontline healthcare services in the public sector: a scoping review of current and future prospects in low and middle-income countries of south and south-east Asia', *BMC Public Health*, 20(880). https://doi.org/10.1186/s12889-020-08975-0

Nandi, A., Hajizadeh, M., Harper, S., Koski, A., Strumpf, E.C. and Heymann, J. (2016), 'Increased duration of paid maternity leave lowers infant mortality in low- and middle-income countries: a quasi-experimental study', *PLoS Medicine*, 13(3), e1001985. https://doi.org/10.1371/journal.pmed.1001985

Narayan, D., Chambers, R., Shah, M.K. and Petesch, P. (2000), *Voices of the Poor: Crying Out for Change*, Oxford University Press for the World Bank, New York. http://hdl.handle.net/10986/13848

Narayan, A., Van der Weide, R., Cojocaru, A., Lakner, C., Redaelli, S., Gerszon Mahler, D., Gupta, N., Ramasubbaiah, R. and Thewissen, S. (2018), *Fair Progress? Economic Mobility across Generations around the World*, World Bank Publications, Washington, DC. www.worldbank.org/en/topic/poverty/publication/fair-progress-economic-mobility-across-generations-around-the-world

Nederlands Jeugdinstituut (2020), 'Kind arme ouders krijgt vaak lager schooladvies', *NJI*, 11 March.

Nguyen, V. (2016), 'Building livelihood resilience in changing climate', Presented at the Asia Regional Conference, Kuala Lumpur, Malaysia. Referenced in S. Hallegatte, M. Bangalore, L. Bonzanigo, M. Fay, T. Kane, U. Narloch, J. Rozenberg, D. Treguer and A. Vogt-Schilb, *Shock Waves: Managing the Impacts of Climate Change on Poverty*, Climate Change and Development Series, World Bank Group, Washington, DC. http://documents.worldbank.org/curated/en/260011486755946625/Shock-waves-managing-the-impacts-of-climate-change-on-poverty

Oberholzer-Gee, F. (2008), 'Nonemployment stigma as rational herding: a field experiment', *Journal of Economic Behavior & Organization*, 65(1), pp 30–40.

Odusanya, I.A. and Akinlo, A.E. (2021), 'Income inequality and population health in sub-Saharan Africa: a test of income inequality-health hypothesis', *Journal of Population and Social Studies*, 29, pp 235–254.

OECD (Organisation for Economic Co-operation and Development) (2011), *Divided We Stand: Why Inequality Keeps Rising*, OECD, Paris.

OECD (2015a), *In It Together: Why Less Inequality Benefits All*, OECD Publishing, Paris. https://doi.org/10.1787/9789264235120-en

OECD (2015b), *Integrating Social Services for Vulnerable Groups: Bridging Sectors for Better Service Delivery*, OECD, Paris. http://dx.doi.org/10.1787/9789264233775-en

OECD (2018a), *A Broken Social Elevator? How to Promote Social Mobility*, OECD, Paris. https://doi.org/10.1787/9789264301085-en

OECD (2018b), *Statistical Insights: New Evidence Shows that Almost 40% of People Are Economically Vulnerable in the OECD*, OECD, Paris. www.oecd.org/sdd/statistical-insights-new-evidence-shows-that-almost-40-of-people-are-economically-vulnerable-in-the-oecd.htm

OECD (2019a), *Society at a Glance 2019: OECD Social Indicators*, OECD Publishing, Paris, https://doi.org/10.1787/soc_glance-2019-en

OECD (2019b), *Changing the Odds for Vulnerable Children: Building Opportunities and Resilience*, OECD Publishing, Paris, https://doi.org/10.1787/a2e8796c-en

OECD (2020a), *Combatting COVID-19's Effect on Children*, OECD, Paris. https://read.oecd-ilibrary.org/view/?ref=132_132643-m91j2scsyh&title=Combatting-COVID19-s-effect-on-children

OECD (2020b), 'Securing the recovery, ambition, and resilience for the well-being of children in the post-COVID-19 Decade', *Webinar paper*, OECD Centre on Well-being, Inclusion, Sustainability and Equal Opportunity (WISE), OECD, Paris. www.oecd.org/social/family/child-well-being/OECD-WISE-Webinar-Children-Post-Covid19-Decade-Oct2020.pdf

OECD (2021a), *Inheritance Taxation in OECD Countries*, OECD, Paris.

OECD (2021b), 'Redistribution from a joint income–wealth perspective: results from 16 European OECD countries', *OECD Social, Employment and Migration Working Papers*, 257, OECD, Paris.

OECD (2022), *Education at a Glance 2022*. www.oecd-ilibrary.org/fr/education/education-at-a-glance-2022_3197152b-en

OECD and European Union (2018), *Health at a Glance: Europe 2018: State of Health in the EU Cycle*, OECD Publishing, Paris; European Union, Brussels. https://doi.org/10.1787/health_glance_eur-2018-en

OHCHR (Office of the High Commissioner for Human Rights) (2005), *Principles and Guidelines for a Human Rights Approach to Poverty Reduction Strategies*, OHCHR, Geneva.

OHCHR (2012), *Guiding Principles on Extreme Poverty and Human Rights*, Human Rights Council resolution 21/11 of 27 September 2012, OHCHR, Geneva. www.ohchr.org/Documents/Publicati ons/OHCHR_ExtremePovertyandHumanRights_EN.pdf

Olsson, L., Opondo, M., Tschakert, P., Agrawal, A., Eriksen, S.H., Ma, S., Perch, L.N. and Zakieldeen, S.A. (2014), 'Livelihoods and poverty', in C.B. Field, V.R. Barros, D.J. Dokken, K.J. Mach, M.D. Mastrandrea, T.E. Bilir, M. Chatterjee, K.L. Ebi, Y.O. Estrada, R.C. Genova, B. Girma, E.S. Kissel, A.N. Levy, S. MacCracken, P.R. Mastrandrea and L.L. White (eds), *Climate Change 2014: Impacts, Adaptation, and Vulnerability. Part A: Global and Sectoral Aspects. Contribution of Working Group II to the Fifth Assessment Report of the Intergovernmental Panel on Climate Change*, Cambridge University Press, Cambridge, UK and New York, pp 793–832.

Omilola, B. and Kaniki, S. (2014), *Social Protection in Africa. A Review of Potential Contribution and Impact on Poverty Reduction,* United Nations Development Program (UNDP), New York.

Ostry, J.D., Berg, A. and Tsangarides, C.G. (2014), 'Redistribution, inequality and growth', *IMF Staff Discussion Note*, International Monetary Fund, Washington, DC.

PACE (Parliamentary Assembly of the Council of Europe) (2015), *Social Services in Europe: Legislation and Practice of the Removal of Children from Their Families in Council of Europe Member States* (Report, Doc. 13730), Council of Europe, Strasbourg.

Parker, S. and Vogl, T. (2018), 'Do conditional cash transfers improve economic outcomes in the next generation? Evidence from Mexico', *National Bureau for Economic Research Working Paper*, 24303.

Pascoe, J.M., Wood, D.L., Duffee J.H. and Kuo, A. (2016), 'Mediators and adverse effects of child poverty in the United States', *Paediatrics*, 137(4), e20160340. https://pediatrics.aappublications. org/content/137/4/e20160340

Paskov M., Gërxhani, K. and Van De Werfhorst, H.G. (2017), 'Giving up on the Joneses? The relationship between income inequality and status-seeking', *European Sociological Review*, 33(1), pp 112–23.

Paul, D. (2021), 'Merging the poverty and environment agendas. Still only one Earth: lessons from 50 years of UN sustainable development policy', *Brief*, 11, International Institute for Sustainable Development (IISD). www.iisd.org/articles/deep-dive/merging-poverty-and-environment-agendas

Peña-Casas, R., Ghailani, D., Spasova, S. and Vanhercke, B. (2019), *In-work Poverty in Europe. A Study of National Policies*, European Social Policy Network (ESPN), Brussels: European Commission.

Peter G. Peterson Foundation (2021), *What Are the Economic Costs of Poverty?* PGDF, New York. www.pgpf.org/blog/2018/09/what-are-the-economic-costs-of-child-poverty

Pettigrew, T.F. and Tropp, L.R. (2000), 'Does intergroup contact reduce prejudice: Recent meta-analytic findings', in S. Oskamp (ed), *Reducing Prejudice and Discrimination*, pp 93–114, Lawrence Erlbaum Associates Publisher, Mahwah.

Phelps, E.S. (1972), 'The statistical theory of racism and sexism', *American Economic Review*, 62(4), pp 659–661.

Phillips, M. (2011), 'Parenting, time use, and disparities in academic outcomes', in G.J. Duncan and R.J. Murnane (eds), *Whither Opportunity? Rising Inequality, Schools, and Children's Life Chances*, pp 207–228, Russell Sage Foundation, New York.

Pickett, K.E. and Wilkinson, R.G. (2015), 'Income inequality and health: a causal review', *Social Science & Medicine*, 128, pp 316–326.

Piketty, T. (2014), *Capital in the Twenty-First Century*, The Belknap Press of Harvard, Cambridge, MA.

Pouw, N., Bender, K., Dipple, L., Schuering, E., Böber, C., Adamba, C. and Alatinga, K. (2017), 'Exploring the interaction effects between two social protection programmes in Ghana: are the poor and extremely poor benefitting?', *SHPIG Working Paper*, EADI, Bonn. https://doi.org/10.13140/RG.2.2.30251.75049

Power, A. (2015), *Sport and Poverty*, Child Poverty Action Group, London. https://cpag.org.uk/sites/default/files/CPAG-Poverty154-Sport-and-poverty-summer2016.pdf

Public Health England (2018), 'Chapter 5: inequalities in health', in *Health Profile for England: 2018*. https://www.gov.uk/government/publications/health-profile-for-england-2018

Putnam, R.D. (2015), *Our Kids. The American Dream in Crisis*, Simon & Schuster, New York.

Ralston, L., Andrews, C. and Hsiao, A. (2017), 'The impacts of safety nets in Africa: what are we learning?', *Policy Research Working Paper*, 8255. World Bank, Washington, DC. https://openknowle dge.worldbank.org/handle/10986/28916

Randstad (2021), *Etude Randstad SmartData sur le marché de l'emploi*, 17 February.

Rao, G. (2019), 'Familiarity does not breed contempt: generosity, discrimination and diversity in Delhi Schools', *American Economic Review*, 109(3), pp 774–809.

Raphael, S. and Winter-Ebmer, R. (2001), 'Identifying the effect of unemployment on crime', *Journal of Law and Economics*, 44(1), pp 259–83.

Ravallion, M. (2009), 'Do poorer countries have less capacity for redistribution?' *Policy Research Working Paper 5046*, Washington DC: World Bank.

Rea, D. and Burton, T. (2019), 'New evidence on the Heckman Curve', *Journal of Economic Surveys*, 34(2), pp 241–262. https:// onlinelibrary.wiley.com/doi/abs/10.1111/joes.12353

Redmond, G., Schnepf, S.V. and Suhrcke, M. (2002), 'Attitudes to inequality after ten years of transition', *Innocenti Working Paper*, 88, UNICEF Innocenti Research Centre, Florence.

Reynolds, L. and Robinson, N. (2005), *Full House? How Overcrowded Housing Affects Families*, Shelter, London.

Reynolds, M.O. and Smolensky, E. (1977), *Public Expenditures, Taxes and the Distribution of Income: The United States, 1950, 1961, 1970*, New York, Academic Press.

Reynolds, R. (2013), 'Glucocorticoid excess and the developmental origins of disease: two decades of testing the hypothesis', *Psychoneuroendocrinology*, 38(1), pp 1–11.

Ribas, R. and Soares, F. (2011), 'Is the effect of conditional transfers on labor supply negligible everywhere?'. http://conference.iza. org/conference_files/worldb2011/ribas_r6802.pdf

Richardson, M. and Hallam, J. (2013), 'Exploring the psychological rewards of a familiar semi-rural landscape: connecting to local nature through a mindful approach', *The Humanistic Psychologist*, 41(1), pp 35–53.

Roex, K.L.A., Huijts, T. and Sieben, I. (2019), 'Attitudes towards income inequality: "winners" versus "losers" of the perceived meritocracy', *Acta Sociologica* 62(1), pp 47–63.

Rohwerder, B. (2014), 'The impact of conflict on poverty', *GSDRC Helpdesk Research Report*, 1118, Governance and Social Development Resource Centre, University of Birmingham, Birmingham. https://assets.publishing.service.gov.uk/media/57a089a5ed915d3cfd000364/hdq1118.pdf

Rosas, N. and Sabarwal, S. (2016), *Public Works as a Productive Safety Net in a Post-Conflict Setting: Evidence from a Randomized Evaluation in Sierra Leone*, World Bank, Washington, DC.

Rothstein, B. and Uslaner, E.M. (2005), 'All for all: equality, corruption, and social trust', *World Politics*, 58(1), pp 41–72.

Rowe, M.L. (2017), 'Understanding socioeconomic differences in parents' speech to children', *Child Development Perspectives*, 12(2), pp 1221–1227.

Sandel, M.J. (2020), *The Tyranny of Merit: What's Become of the Common Good?* Allen Lane, London.

Sanfilippo, M., Martorano, B. and De Neubourg, C. (2012), 'The impact of social protection on children: a review of the literature', *Innocenti Working Papers*, 2012–06, UNICEF, Rome.

Save the Children (2016), *Ending Educational and Child Poverty in Europe*, Save the Children, Brussels. www.savethechildren.nl/sci-nl/media/Save-the-children/PDF/ending_educational_and_child_poverty_in_europe_02-12-2016.pdf

Save the Children (2020a), *The Effectiveness of Cash Transfer Programming for Children*, Save the Children, London. https://resourcecentre.savethechildren.net/node/17552/pdf/Save%20the%20Children%20Cash%20Transfers%20Evidence%20Summary%20-%202%20Pager.pdf

Save the Children (2020b), *Scoping and Sector Review of Social Protection in Somaliland*, Save the Children, London. https://resourcecen tre.savethechildren.net/node/17845/pdf/scoping_and_sector_ review_of_social_protection_in_somaliland.pdf

Save the Children (2020c), *Universal Child Benefits (UCBs): A Foundation to End Child Poverty*, Save the Children, London.

Scitovsky, T. (1992 [1976]), *The Joyless Economy. The Psychology of Human Satisfaction*, Oxford University Press, Oxford and New York.

Scott, L. (2006), 'Chronic poverty and the environment: a vulnerability perspective', *Working Paper*, 62, Chronic Poverty Research Centre. www.odi.org/sites/odi.org.uk/files/odi-assets/ publications-opinion-files/3429.pdf

Sen, A.K. (1997), 'Inequality, unemployment and contemporary Europe', *International Labour Review* 136(2), pp 155–171.

Sepulveda Carmona, M. (2014), *Report of the Special Rapporteur on Extreme Poverty and Human Rights, Presented at the 26th Session of the Human Rights Council* (A/HRC/26/28) (22 May).

Shiferaw, B., Tesfaye, K., Kassie, M., Abate, T., Prasanna, B.M. and Menkir, A. (2014), 'Managing vulnerability to drought and enhancing livelihood resilience in sub-Saharan Africa: technological, institutional and policy options', *Weather and Climate Extremes*, 3, pp 67–79. https://doi.org/10.1016/j.wace.2014.04.004

Singh, G.K. and Lee, H. (2021), 'Marked disparities in life expectancy by education, poverty level, occupation and housing tenure in the United States, 1997–2014', *International Journal of MCH and AIDS*, 10(1), pp 7–18.

Soares, S., Guerreiro Osório, R., Veras Soares, F., Medeiros, M. and Zepeda, E. (2007), 'Conditional cash transfers in Brazil, Chile and Mexico: implications for inequality', *Working Paper* 35, International Poverty Centre, United Nations Development Programme, Brasilia.

Social Protection Committee (2022a), *Portfolio of EU Social Indicators for the Monitoring of Progress towards the EU Objectives for Social Protection and Social Inclusion (2022 Update)*, European Commission, Brussels. https://ec.europa.eu/social/main.jsp?catId=738&lan gId=en&pubId=8513&furtherPubs=yes

Social Protection Committee (2022b), *Social Protection Committee Annual Report 2022: Review of the Social Protection Performance Monitor (SPPM) and Developments in Social Protection Policies*, European Commission, Brussels. https://ec.europa.eu/social/BlobServlet?docId=26193&langId=en

Solnick, S. and Hemenway, D. (1998), 'Is more always better? A survey on positional concerns', *Journal of Economic Behavior & Organization*, 37(3), pp 373–383.

Sornarajah, M. (1986), 'State responsibility and bilateral investment treaties', *Journal of World Trade Law*, 20, pp 79–98.

Steele, C.M. and Aronson, J. (1995), 'Stereotype threat and the intellectual test performance of African Americans', *Journal of Personality and Social Psychology*, 69(5), pp 797–811.

Sullivan, K.M. (1986), 'Sins of discrimination: last term's affirmative action cases', *Harvard Law Review*, 100, pp 78–98.

Sumner, K. and Kusumaningrum, S. (2015), *AIPJ Baseline Study on Legal Identity Indonesia's Missing Millions*. https://getinthepicture.org/resource/aipj-baseline-study-legal-identity-indonesias-missing-millions

Tcherneva, P.R. (2019), 'The federal job guarantee: prevention, not just a cure', *Challenge*, 62(4), pp 253–272.

Tcherneva, P.R. (2020), *The Case for a Job Guarantee*, Polity, Cambridge, UK.

The Lancet (2020), 'A future for the world's children? A WHO–UNICEF–Lancet commission', *The Lancet Commissions*, 395. www.thelancet.com/pdfs/journals/lancet/PIIS0140-6736(19)32540-1.pdf

Thévenon, O. and Edmonds, E. (2019), 'Child labour: causes, consequences and policies to tackle it', *Working Papers*, 235, OECD, Paris. www.oecd-ilibrary.org/social-issues-migration-health/child-labour_f6883e26-en

Thornton, M. (2018), 'Social status: the last bastion of discrimination', *Anti-Discrimination Law Review*, 1(3), pp 1–26.

Tunstall, R. Bevan, M., Bradshaw, J., Croucher, K., Duffy, S., Hunter, C., Jones, A., Rugg, J., Wallace, A. and Wilcox, S. (2013), *How Housing Can Mitigate or Exacerbate the Impact of Poverty on People's Lives*, Joseph Rowntree Foundation, York. www.jrf.org.uk/report/links-between-housing-and-poverty

UNDP (United Nations Development Programme) (2022), *Addressing the Cost of Living Crisis in Vulnerable Countries*, United Nations High-Level Political Forum on Sustainable Development (HLPF).

UNDP, SUSSC (Special Unit for South-South Cooperation) and ILO (2011), *Sharing Innovating Experiences, vol. 18: Successful Social Protection Floor Experiences*, UNDP, New York.

UNESCO (United Nations Educational, Scientific and Cultural Organization) (2020), *Global Education Monitoring Report 2020: Inclusion and Education: All Means All.* UNESCO, Paris.

UNICEF (United Nations International Children's Emergency Fund) (2016), *The State of the World's Children 2016: A Fair Chance for Every Child*, UNICEF, New York. www.unicef.org/reports/state-worlds-children-2016

UNICEF (2020), *Averting a Lost COVID Generation: A Six-point Plan to Respond, Recover and Reimagine a Post-Pandemic World for Every Child*, UNICEF, New York. www.unicef.org/media/86881/file/Averting-a-lost-covid-generation-world-childrens-day-data-and-advocacy-brief-2020.pdf

UNICEF and the Global Coalition to End Child Poverty (2017), *A World Free from Child Poverty: A Guide to the Task to Achieve the Vision*, UNICEF, New York. www.unicef.org/reports/world-free-child-poverty

United Nations (2015), Sustainable Development Goals.

United Nations (2022), *Sustainable Development Goals Report.* https://unstats.un.org/sdgs/report/2022/The-Sustainable-Development-Goals-Report-2022.pdf

United Nations Economic and Social Council (2015), 'Everyone counts: ensuring a response of official statistics to Sustainable Development Goals consistent with human rights', *Note by the United Nations Office of the High Commissioner for Human Rights (OHCHR)*, UN doc. ECE/CES/2015/35 (8 May 2015). www.ohchr.org/en/documents/tools-and-resources/everyone-counts-ensuring-response-official-statistics-sustainable

United Nations Economic and Social Council (2020), 'Affordable housing and social protection systems for all to address homelessness', *Resolution adopted by the Economic and Social Council on 18 June 2020*, E/RES/2020/7. https://digitallibrary.un.org/record/3869551/files/E_RES_2020_7-EN.pdf?ln=en

United Nations General Assembly (2005), *The Centrality of Employment to Poverty Eradication*, Report of the Secretary-General, A/60/314.

UN Committee on Economic, Social and Cultural Rights (2001), 'Poverty and the International Covenant on Economic, Social and Cultural Rights', *Statement adopted on 4 May 2001*, UN doc. E/C.12/2001/10 (10 May 2001). https://www2.ohchr.org/english/bodies/cescr/docs/statements/E.C.12.2001.10Poverty-2001.pdf

UN Committee on Economic, Social and Cultural Rights (2009), *General Comment No. 20: Non-discrimination in Economic, Social and Cultural Rights*, E/C.12/GC/20 (2 July 2009), Geneva

UN Committee on Economic, Social and Cultural Rights (2016), Statement adopted by the Committee, *Public Debt, Austerity Measures and the International Covenant on Economic, Social and Cultural Rights*, E/C.12/2016/1 (24 June 2016), Geneva.

Uslaner, E.M. and Brown, M. (2005), 'Inequality, trust, and civic engagement', *American Politics Research*, 33(6), pp 868–894.

Van Belle, E., Di Stasio, V., Caers, R., De Couck, M. and Baert, S. (2018), 'Why are employers put off by long spells of unemployment?' *European Sociological Review*, 34(6), pp 694–710.

van Ham, M., Hedman, L., Manley, D., Coulter, R. and Östh, J. (2014), 'Intergenerational transmission of neighbourhood poverty: an analysis of neighbourhood histories of individuals', *Transactions of the Institute of British Geographers*, 39(3), pp 402–417. https://rgs-ibg.onlinelibrary.wiley.com/doi/10.1111/tran.12040

van Parijs, P. and Vanderborght, Y. (2017), *Basic Income: A Radical Proposal for a Free Society and a Sane Economy*, Harvard University Press, Cambridge, MA and London.

Veblen, T. (1899), *The Theory of the Leisure Class: An Economic Study in the Evolution of Institutions*, Macmillan, New York.

Veltman, A. (2016), *Meaningful Work*, Oxford University Press, Oxford.

Veras Soares, F., Perez Ribas, R. and Issamu Hirata, G. (2008), *Los Logros y las Carencias de las Transferencias de Efectivo Condicionadas. Evaluación del Impacto del Programa Tekoporã del Paraguay* (*Achievements and Shortfalls of Conditional Cash Transfers: Impact Evaluation of Paraguay's Tekoporã Programme*), International Policy Centre for Inclusive Growth, Brasilia.

Wagmiller, R. and Adelman, R. (2009), *Childhood and Intergenerational Poverty: The Long-Term Consequences of Growing Up Poor*, National Centre for Children in Poverty, New York. www.nccp.org/wp-content/uploads/2020/05/text_909.pdf

Waldfogel, H.B, Sheehy-Skeffington, J., Hauser, O. and Kteily, N.S. (2021), 'Ideology selectively shapes attention to inequality', *Proceedings of the National Academy of Sciences*, 118(14), e2023985118.

Walker, R. (2014), *The Shame of Poverty*, Oxford University Press, Oxford.

Watts, M.J. and Mitchell, W.F. (2000), 'The costs of unemployment in Australia', *The Economic and Labour Relations Review*, 11(2), pp 180–197.

WHO (World Health Organization) (2021), 'Malnutrition', *Factsheet*. www.who.int/news-room/fact-sheets/detail/malnutrition

WHO and IBRD (International Bank for Reconstruction and Development)/The World Bank (2017), *Tracking Universal Health Coverage: 2017 Global Monitoring Report*, WHO, Geneva.

Wilkinson, R. and Pickett, K. (2018), *The Inner Level: How More Equal Societies Reduce Stress, Restore Sanity and Improve Everyone's Well-being*, Allen Lane, London.

World Bank (2018), *Learning to Realize Education's Promise*, The World Bank, Washington, DC. www.worldbank.org/en/publication/wdr2018

REFERENCES

World Food Programme (2022), *Global Report on Food Crises – 2022*, Global Network Against Food Crises and Food Security Information Network. www.wfp.org/publications/global-rep ort-food-crises-2022

World Inequality Database (nd), https://wid.world/

Yoshida, N., Narayan, A. and Wu, H. (2020), 'How COVID-19 affects households in poorest countries: insights from phone surveys', *World Bank Blogs*, 10 December. https://blogs.worldb ank.org/voices/how-covid-19-affects-households-poorest-countr ies-insights-phone-surveys

Young Lives (2008), *Department of International Development*, University of Oxford, Oxford. www.younglives.org.uk

Ziol-Guest, K.M., Duncan, G.J., Kalil, A. and Boyce, W.T. (2012), 'Early childhood poverty, immune-mediated disease processes, and adult productivity', *Proceedings of the National Academy of Sciences of the United States of America*, 109 Suppl 2, pp 17289–17293. https://doi.org/10.1073/pnas.1203167109

Index

References to figures appear in *italic* type. References to footnotes show both the page number and the note number (12n2).

UNICEF *see* United Nations
    International Children's
    Emergency Fund
United Kingdom (UK) 54, 69
  England 21
  Scotland 125
United Nations Development
    Programme (UNDP) 13–14
United Nations Educational,
    Scientific and Cultural
    Organization (UNESCO) 35,
    37, 105
United Nations International
    Children's Emergency
    Fund 13, 23, 26, 39, 47,
    69, 89
United States (US)
  child poverty 2, 12, 13, 69
  discrimination 47–48
  early childhood education
      and care (ECEC) 35,
      100–101
  employment opportunities 44
  inheritance tax 119
  inter-generational
      mobility 32–33
  life expectancy 20, 64
  redistribution 141–142
  school expenditure 36
  wealth inequality 16
universal basic income
    (UBI) 117–119
universalism, progressive 102,
    139–142
US *see* United States (US)

V

value added tax (VAT) 80,
    87–88, 88n3
VAT *see* value added tax (VAT)
vicious cycle 2, 5, 13, 20, 28, 48,
    49–50, 58, 67, 75, 100, 130,
    134, 142, 148, 156

W

wage 99, 100, 117
  see also living wage;
      minimum wage
wage earners 80, 88
wasting 13, 25, 26
wealth inequality 16, 66–68, 82,
    118–119
wealth tax 82
WHO *see* World Health
    Organization (WHO)
women 53, 54, 97–98
work, right to 112–117
World Bank 1, 4, 80, 151
World Health Organization
    (WHO) 26, 28

Y

young adults, basic income
    for 117–119

Z

Zambia 93, 94
Zimbabwe 93